LIVING
with PAIN
without
Becoming
ONE

Craig Selness

WORTHY®
Inspired

Library of Congress Control Number: 2017943806

To Brenda

---

*Who has loved me, fought for me, comforted me,
inspired me, cared for me and prayed for me.
I am grateful, and honored, to be called your husband.*

CONTENTS

FOREWORD

by John Ortberg

Pain, as Dr. Paul Brand said long ago, is the gift nobody wants. It alerts us to what has gone wrong in our bodies or possibly our lives. The inability to experience pain is itself a crippling problem for human beings.

But . . .

Pain is the bane of human existence. It can cause people to wonder whether life is worth continuing. It can damage our ability to love others. It can keep us relentlessly focused on our own condition. It can smother all the joy and wonder out of life. It can turn prayer into ashes, faith into despair; it can drive us to our knees or keep us from them.

Craig Selness understands about pain. Partly this is because he is a pastor. He has been educated (by the way—he's got a law degree, too, so he's already lots of IQ points ahead of most of us) to think clearly about how a good God and a pain-filled life can fit together. He has sat by the bedsides of suffering and dying people.

But he has also faced more than his share of pain. I'll let him tell that story. But I get to work alongside him in the church world, and I see how he cares for people and patiently deals with a level of physical suffering that would send most of us looking for cheap and easy ways to escape.

Living with Pain without Becoming One is the guide you have been looking for. It is deeply immersed in the text of Scripture. The Bible itself is, among other things, a book about pain. Job may be the single most famous paragon of unexplained suffering in human literature. More than that, Craig helps locate the mystery of suffering—and its ultimate meaning and redemption—in the cross of Jesus. It is there that we meet what no mere human being could have predicted—the suffering God. We may never know on this side of the curtain why it is that our world is filled with so much suffering. But we meet at the cross a God who cares about suffering with measureless compassion. And in that shared suffering comes a hope that the mere cessation of pain cannot provide.

If you have picked up this book there is a good chance that you, or someone you dearly loved, is deeply troubled by the problem of pain. I hope that in these pages you are met by help and help. I hope your story is just a few thoughts away from a whole new chapter. I hope Craig becomes your guide and friend through the maze of pain.

"When the pain *is* me:
Wanting to be better even when
I don't feel better."

CHAPTER ONE

So you're in pain. People can see it in your face. You don't talk about it all the time, but it hurts pretty much all the time. And you're not alone. As of 2017, there are over 324 million people who live in the United States, and *100 million* of us report that our pain is chronic. That's more than the number of people who suffer from diabetes, heart disease, and cancer . . . *combined.* The annual cost of treating our pain, plus the economic costs related to lost productivity? Over $600 billion.[1] As evidence of the epidemic chronic pain has become, it's been reported that in 2015 there were more prescriptions written for pain killers in multiple states, including Alabama, Tennessee, and West Virginia, than there were people living in those states.[2]

And then there's this cost to factor in—chronic pain can shrink our brains and shorten our lives. A study conducted at Northwestern University in 2004 reported that chronic pain can reduce the volume of our brain tissue by as much as 11 percent and age us 10 to 20 years.[3] It doesn't seem fair that the payoff for all our pain is to get a smaller brain and the fast track to senility, does it?

If you suffer with chronic pain, you know how all-consuming it can be. Sometimes you don't care as much about what time it is as you do about when you can take the next something—anything—for your pain. You may measure how long you can be away from your house by how long it will take for your ice pack to melt. It's often the last thing you think about at night and—if the pain gives you permission to fall asleep—it'll be the first thing you think about in the morning.

And, as many pain sufferers have pointed out, one of the frustrations is that pain is quite often an "invisible illness." People see nothing out of the ordinary; you look perfectly healthy. You probably aren't in a cast or wheelchair, and you aren't bleeding. Yet you still hurt, and you would very much appreciate some sympathy. But how can you let people know just how much you hurt without sounding like, well, a whiner?

For most of us—those who have the good fortune of being loved by family and friends—what can be most troubling about our pain is not necessarily the physical misery or the price of pain meds. It is, instead, *who we become.* What is particularly disturbing to us is when we realize not only that we're *in* constant pain, but that we have *become* a pain to the people we love . . . and that we have become a pain even to ourselves.

I was sure that would never happen to me. I was confident I could and would rise above any pain or suffering that might come my way, that pain would only make me stronger and better and an inspiration to one and all, that songs would be written and stories told about how I turned my scars into stars and my bruises into blessings.

Or maybe not.

For most of my life, pain wasn't an issue. I prided myself on my high pain threshold. I once scolded my young children for bleeding all over our kitchen floor, only to have my wife point out that *I* was the one causing the mess. I'd had no idea I was bleeding or how I cut myself (it might have been the chain saw, but that's another story). The point is that I simply didn't feel the pain. I had, of course, *seen* pain often, particularly in my wife—childbirth times three and the pain of a herniated disc with an ensuing surgery. And as a pastor I had prayed with people in pain of all kinds—physical pain, the pain of betrayal and divorce, the pain of being fired, the pain of losing a lifelong spouse . . .

Sure, I knew what it felt like to hurt (I assure you, the kidney stones got my full attention). But I was confident I could handle any pain that came my way, even better than most. I could "gut" through it, I thought. I would recite Bible verses to myself. I was a man—a Norwegian man, at that; we don't show emotion, and we don't give an inch to pain. Pain is unpleasant, certainly. It's a nuisance. But my experience in playing athletics had convinced me that my coaches were right: one way or another, there was no pain I could not simply play through. I subscribed to the motto "Pain is weakness leaving the body." So if I'm hurting, it only means I'm getting stronger.

Then, at the age of 54, I was diagnosed with necrosis in my left hip—the blood had stopped flowing to my hip, and the bone was dying. Actually, my hip hurt for over a year even before I went to a doctor; I just assumed the pain would go away. Then the surgeries to address the problem began, a total of five in thirteen months.

And I was surprised at how poorly I handled the pain.

My first clue that I was not the "pain warrior" I thought I was came the day of my second hip surgery, the day of my doctor's first attempt at a total hip replacement. A good friend of mine from our church, who'd had a hip replacement when he was significantly older than me (and both knees replaced too), assured me that he had very little pain following his surgery. My doctor also told me that since I was relatively young and had kept in good shape, I should bounce back fairly quickly. But when I woke up from surgery, I was in pain . . . pain far more severe than anything I had yet experienced. When the doctor visited me that afternoon, he expressed mild surprise at my pain and ordered more pain medication. It didn't help. My friend Joe—the one with the hip replacement, no problems, minimal pain, and *no* pain after day eleven—came to visit me. He sat with me for a time, encouraged me, sympathized with me. He was being a pastor to me, even though I was his pastor. And while he sat with me, I looked him in the eyes and said with all seriousness, and in a bit of an accusatory tone, "You lied to me! This is miserable. Why would you tell me it wasn't going to be bad?"

What kind of pastor calls one of his elderly members, one of his good friends, a liar? I began to realize that things were not going to go as I had assumed they would.

My second clue came on Christmas. The hip replacement had taken place four days earlier—not the best timing to celebrate the holidays with family. My wife made my favorite meal for dinner, but the smell of the roasted meat made me nauseated. We opened presents, and after a bit I felt the need to lie down. My wife and son helped me lug my swollen leg to the family room. But within minutes of getting settled on the couch, I started to cry. Big tears. Loudly. I had no idea why I was crying; I didn't have a lot of personal experience with tears. Yes, I had cried when we put down our two golden retrievers—I do have a heart, after all. But in our thirty-plus years of marriage, my wife had seen me cry, at most, a mere handful of times. And as I wept that day, the thought came to me, "Maybe I'm not as good at this pain thing as I thought." (Jonathan Rottenberg, an emotion researcher from the University of South Florida, offers an explanation for tears like these: "Crying signals to yourself and other people that there's some important problem that is at least temporarily beyond your ability to cope.")[4]

The clincher came some months later, after the fifth surgery on my hip when a fifth surgeon went in to revise the original hip replacement that had gone so badly nine months earlier. I had been quite miserable during the whole process. I dropped from 162 pounds to somewhere in the 130s, and the doctors weren't sure why. The fifth surgery, while it fixed some problems, actually caused more issues, making me sicker than before and causing some significant nerve damage in my foot, leg, and back. My wife could not have been stronger or kinder through it all. Like me, Brenda has a strong faith in God. She believes God works everything together for good; she believes in the power of prayer; she believes God gives us the grace to handle every hardship.

But this was my final clue that I was not as brave or as strong a patient as I believed I was, that I was not handling my pain as well as I had in the past. One evening Brenda and I were talking about what we were praying for and asking God to do. And my wife said this, with all sincerity and tenderness: "I told God that if He wasn't going to heal you, then He should take you." She wasn't being mean when she said this. She wasn't angry at God or bitter toward God. But it occurred to me that if my wife was giving God permission to "take" her husband, then maybe (once again) I wasn't handling my pain all that well.

Yes, I was in pain . . . a whole lot of pain. But more than that, I realized this inconvenient truth: *I had become a pain.*

That's not what Brenda said. She never once told me that I needed to have a better attitude or that I should be stronger or more gracious. To the contrary, she only told me that she was proud of how I was handling the whole ordeal. But God was using my wife to gently point out that while I was trying my best to manage my pain well, I had, in fact, become something of a pain to the people who loved me the most. And a corollary truth dawned on me: *I had become a pain to me.* I did not like who I had become during my trial. I did not like the way I had allowed the pain to dominate my thoughts and dictate my feelings. I was not happy about being in pain, but even more so, I was not happy about the *me* I had allowed myself to become.

Have you ever had a moment like that, where a close friend or a partner pulled you aside and pointed out that you had become a bit of a pain? Yes, they appreciate how hard you're trying; they recognize that they don't completely understand what you're going through. But because they love you, they want you to know . . . you can be better than how you've been, even in your pain.

Or maybe it wasn't something someone said to you—it was what they didn't say. It was the look in their eyes when you barked at the salesman or the quick exit that occurred when it became clear that nothing they said would change your mood. When did you realize that *you* had become a pain?

WHEN PAIN PREDOMINATES

My physical pain is better now, but it has never gone away. It's quite possible—in fact, very likely—that it will never go away, that pain is now my predominant state of being. It is that way for so many people, I've learned. I saw a poster once with this inspiring sentiment: "H.O.P.E.: Hold On, Pain Ends." Only sometimes it doesn't.

My oldest brother, while driving a motorcycle, got hit by a truck that ran a red light, and he had to have his lower left leg amputated when he was in his twenties. Obviously, legs don't grow back, and while his pain has improved significantly, he always has some level of pain. A woman in our church has fibromyalgia. She is always in pain, to some degree or another. The daughter who was told by her parents (in their last conversation before the parents' passing), "We should have had an abortion"—that's a hurt that hangs on. It can be the regret we feel over a poor life choice, sticking like Velcro. There are some injuries that cause acute pain and then heal with time. There are other injuries—physical or emotional—that change us. The pain changes how we think and feel, how we sleep or wake up. We don't "get back to normal." Our pain adheres to us like an unfortunate tattoo.

Every one of us learned as a child that pain is inevitable. None of us would ever choose to live in pain; in fact, we do most everything we can to avoid it. But the pain-free life is simply not an option in this world. Life begins with pain—it certainly did for your mother—and it often ends with pain. In between? Bruises, wounds, broken hearts, unfulfilled dreams, repeated surgeries, lingering illnesses, and relationships gone awry. No, it's not all painful. Much of life is filled with joy and laughter, good food and friends. But pain . . . well, in one way or another, it just won't leave us alone.

So here's the question, one I've spent quite a bit of time contemplating since hearing my wife's prayer for me—*How do I live with pain without becoming one?*

WHEN THE PAIN IS YOU

Let me paint a picture of someone whose pain has made them a pain. See if this rings any proverbial bells for you. This person cannot get through any conversation, no matter how short, without telling you about their pain. If you try to sympathize with this person by describing a time when *you* were in pain, his or her response will be to tell you how your pain pales in comparison to theirs. "You simply don't know what you're talking about," they say. This person can be a living thesaurus when it comes to describing their sufferings. Their headache doesn't just "hurt"; it's "throbbing" and "stabbing" and "blinding." It's not that they feel "sore"—they are "in anguish," "tortured," "in agony"; their pain is "excruciating." They are "racked" with pain; they have pain "spasms." If this is a person who has had a number of surgeries like me, he or she will be able to tell you the date of every surgery, how long each hospital stay was, what meds they had to take and for how long, and the number of scars present if you just give them a minute to look around and count them all up (actually, that's not true—they've been counted a hundred times).

You don't need me to tell you that it's a pain to be around someone like that. And the reason I know—as I've already confessed—is because I've been a person like that.

But that's not who I want to be.

I don't want to be the kind of person who drives away the people who care about me, the very people I need the most.

Did you ever see the TV show *House*? (It aired from 2004–2012.) Dr. Gregory House, played by Hugh Laurie, was a brilliant doctor and diagnostician. But he lived in chronic pain and used his pain as an excuse to treat people—especially the people who cared about him—with sarcasm, indifference, and even contempt. He lived in pain and managed it by becoming an even bigger pain to every patient and every person who tried to be his friend.

LIVING IN PAIN AND LIVING WELL

I've been a lifelong student of the Bible, and I discovered a long time ago that the Bible has a great deal to say on the subject of pain. It doesn't answer all my questions, by any means, but I'm learning that it tells me everything I really need to know about how to manage pain. For example, 1 Peter is a relatively short book near the end of the New Testament that was written to people who were undergoing a great deal of suffering and hardship. The first readers of this letter lived with a significant degree of pain. And in wondering how to live with pain without becoming one, I was particularly struck with this particular word of challenge: "So then, those who suffer according to God's will should commit themselves to their faithful Creator and continue to do good" (1 Peter 4:19).

That one verse alone taught me two very important truths about pain. First, some pain is part of God's plan for us. It's not an accident; it's not a mistake. *Some of our pain is by divine design.*

Not all of it, of course. In fact, one of the ways the Bible helps us live with pain is by candidly clarifying that there's no all-encompassing answer to the question "Why is this happening to me?" Sometimes my pain is my own fault, and sometimes I'm the victim. Sometimes pain is part of my calling as a Christian, and sometimes it's just plain evil. Fortunately, as we'll see later, the Bible has something helpful to say about how to live with all our pain, no matter where it comes from.

And second, 1 Peter 4:19 tells me that it's our calling as Christians to "continue to do good" even while we suffer. *Suffering doesn't give us a free pass to behave badly.* It is possible to suffer without being insufferable. No, I don't think God expects people to be at their very best when the chemotherapy makes them feel as if someone is trying to pull their throat through their mouth. And there's not a thing in the world wrong with crying or moaning or curling up in a ball while in pain (the Bible has a whole book about this, appropriately titled "Lamentations"). But it is possible, the Bible tells us, to live with pain without becoming one. It is possible to feel miserable and yet "continue to do good."

I was watching the nightly news recently. It was one of those days when all the news was bad news, when the world seemed as if it was coming apart at the seams. A plane had been shot down. A school in the Middle East was mistakenly bombed, killing innocent children and aid workers. No one in Congress could seem to agree on anything. A fire in the state of Washington—the worst fire in Central Washington's history—destroyed hundreds of homes.

But before signing off, the broadcaster wanted us to meet a particular couple, a middle-aged couple who'd just lost their home. This couple had three relatives who lived nearby—and their homes had all burned down as well. But before this couple went to sift through the smoldering ruins of their destroyed residence, they went to a makeshift feeding station. Not to eat. Not to rest. They went there to spend the entire day cooking and serving meals to their neighbors. And they weren't the only residents of Pateros, Washington, who rose to the challenge. As one elderly woman whose home was in ashes said, "There's a time for crying, and there's a time for doing."[5]

Yes, there is a time for crying. Sometimes it hurts so badly, that's pretty much all you can do. But there's also a time for doing, to "continue to do good." Maybe we can't do the good we did before, but we can still do good. We can send an encouraging text; we can give a ride to someone stuck at home; we can watch our neighbors' kids; we can sponsor a needy child; we can let our friends know we're praying for them every day. It takes a bit more energy to do good when we're hurting, and we "feel like it" a little less often than before, but the truth is, "We are God's handiwork, created in Christ Jesus to do good works" (Ephesians 2:10). And even though the pain lingers, nothing is more satisfying than doing what you were made to do.

A Prayer Less Prayed

This quote is attributed to President Kennedy: "Do not pray for easy lives. Pray to be stronger men." I don't keep track of such things, but I suspect I have prayed far more often for God to make my life easier than I have for Him to make me stronger—that I've asked Him to take away my pain far more frequently than I've asked Him to make me better able to manage my pain. In my life, at least, this has been a prayer less prayed.

I've read—devoured, actually—scores of books on pain. One

of my favorites is *Walking with God Through Pain and Suffering* by Pastor Timothy Keller, which includes in each chapter a short testimony of someone who is in the middle of a particularly difficult situation. One story hit home for me. I read it just one day after I tried to play some basketball in my backyard, a hobby that for many years was one of the great joys of my life. It had quickly became painfully apparent that, given the condition of my hip, playing basketball—even just standing and shooting—was no longer an option for me. And the frustration I've felt over the last few years over being "taken out of the game" by my hip surgeries and the resulting nerve damage made me feel particularly gloomy for a time.

The next day I read Pastor Keller's chapter entitled "Learning to Walk," and at the end of the chapter was a short testimony by Mark and Martha, who had four children and had been married for twenty-five years when Mark was diagnosed with ALS. Mark had always been a physically active person, an athlete who cherished being "in the game." Within months of his diagnosis, the only thing Mark could move was his eyes. But sitting at a computer that was able to capture eye movements, Mark wrote this paragraph—and it hit me between the eyes:

> I played sports in my younger years, and I always hated sitting on the bench. One day after my diagnosis, I cried out to God that I thought I was being pulled out of the game when I still had something to offer. His response was, "You have been on the sidelines for some time; you are just now going in the game."[6]

My physical limitations and pain pale in comparison to Mark's; frankly, there is no comparison. But I relate to the feeling of being benched when I still want to be in the game. And the good news is this: In a very real way, God just put me in. It's very possible that you know exactly what I'm talking about, because in the last days, months, and years God has put you in the game too. And I suspect the only way I'm going to do well in this game is by praying a prayer that up until now has been, for me, a prayer less prayed: "God, make me a stronger man." And here's what I believe, what I encourage you to believe: He will. He will give me the strength to continue to do good even when it hurts, to be a better person even when I don't feel better; He will give me the grace to live with my pain without becoming one.

It's time to figure out just what that means.

"When the pain persists:
Managing my pain
by managing my life."

CHAPTER TWO

———

There are two truths about pain I've not been eager to embrace. The first truth is this: *pain is a good and necessary gift from God.* That doesn't sound right, does it—pain a gift? Pain—necessary? It certainly doesn't feel right, not when you're in pain. But once we think about it, we realize that it is inarguably true. There is an upside to pain.

IN PRAISE OF PAIN

Do you remember the first time you put your hand on a hot stove, grabbed a scalding pan, or received a burn another way? To say the least, it hurt. And because it hurt, you took action—action that spared your body more injury. When pain discourages us from doing things that threaten our well-being and survival, it is most definitely our friend.

Or how about this . . . Did you ever have an injury and found yourself avoiding certain normal activities because you were afraid you might cause yourself more pain? Pain—the fear of more pain—motivated you to stay put so your body could heal more quickly and properly.

Maybe you've heard someone talk about the "problem" of pain. It's a reason people sometimes give for not believing in God, as in, "If God is good and loving and all-powerful, then why do people suffer?" And while that is a question deserving a thoughtful, caring, and humble response, the fact is that while the presence of pain in our world might be a knotty philosophical problem, *the absence of pain would be just as much a puzzler.* Then the question would be, "If God is good and loving and all-powerful, then why don't we feel pain when something is wrong?"

When we hurt physically, our bodies are giving us a message— something is needing attention. When a tooth hurts, it means there's a problem with the tooth or the root and we need to go to the dentist. Without that pain we'd simply ignore the decay or infection and end up seriously ill. We have pain to thank for saving our teeth and even our lives.

And it works the same way with our souls. Do you ever feel guilty? Guilt is painful. So is shame. So is regret. And quite often that's a *good* thing. When we do something morally wrong, when we cheat or steal or lie, the pain we feel is a sign that we're still healthy human beings. There are names we give to people who don't feel pain when they willfully do harm to others—like "psychopath," for one. A psychopath is not a healthy person or the kind of person anyone aspires to be. A psychopath is identified in the *Diagnostic and Statistical Manual of Mental Disorders, Fifth Edition* ("DSM-5") as a person having an "antisocial personality disorder," a person without a conscience. Guilt and shame are gifts from God to inform us that something is wrong in our hearts or in our relationships and it needs to be fixed. No one enjoys feeling guilty, but thank God we're healthy enough that our guilt still causes us pain.

Pope Francis, in a Mass given on the Feast of St. Ignatius in 2013, prayed that he and his fellow Jesuits would receive "the grace of shame" for their failures.[1] Guilt and shame over wrongs we've done are gifts of grace from God that motivate us to seek God's forgiveness and the forgiveness of those we've injured. As Paul puts it, "Godly sorrow brings repentance that leads to salvation and leaves no regret" (2 Corinthians 7:10). Modern psychology, as well, acknowledges that guilt and shame often motivate us to make positive changes in our lives and that there can be a benefit to psychological pain.[2] Certainly guilt and shame can be destructive, and they often are. But when the pain of guilt over something I did to betray a friend's trust motivates me to repair that relationship, then the pain of my guilt is surely a gift of grace.

In my years as a pastor I've counseled many couples whose marriages have been upended by broken trust. I was with one couple at the very moment when the wife admitted she had been having an affair with her husband's coworker. She spit out her confession with anger and a bit of pride; when I left their home later that night, I gave the marriage very little chance of survival. But while the wife didn't want to pursue counseling or reconciliation, the husband wasn't ready to quit; he asked me to keep meeting with him to pray for his wife and their future. So we did. We didn't use these words, but we most definitely prayed that God would bless his wife with the "grace of shame." And while it took over a year, God's painful grace prevailed and that couple reunited. Twenty years later, they're still together and thriving as a couple.

So there are times when it's appropriate to thank God for the annoying alarm of pain and to pay close attention to how God might want to use it for your good. Consider whether God has gifted you with pain to show you that there's something wrong in your life—something wrong with your body, your soul, your relationships, or something you can act to rectify. No, pain is not always our friend; it's not usually our friend. But there are times in life when it's the best gift God could give us.

WHEN PAIN PERSISTS

But here's the second truth about pain that I have been slow to embrace—*sometimes the pain doesn't go away.* Not even when you fix the problem.

It makes no sense. If pain tells me there's a problem that needs to be fixed and I fix the problem, the pain should go away, right? Usually it does. My kidney stones caused me significant pain, but once they passed, the pain went away. That's how it's supposed to work. Pain alerts us to an issue, we deal with the issue, the injury heals, and the pain goes away.

Except when it doesn't.

There's a branch of medical science called pain management that exists because of this reality of lingering pain. Medicine treats our injury and pathology to support our healing along with treating our pain to relieve suffering during the healing process. But when a painful injury or pathology is resistant to treatment and persists—when pain persists even after the injury or pathology has healed and when medical science, in fact, cannot identify the cause of the continuing pain—the task of medicine then becomes to help the patient *manage the pain.*[3]

The first time I remember someone talking to me about "pain management" was shortly before my first hip surgery. I didn't pay much attention—after all, I was confident I'd be able to handle any pain that came my way, plus I assumed that whatever pain I was going to experience would be temporary. Fortunately, my wife took notes . . . just in case. She filled my prescription for pain meds. She bought an ice machine—even though I told her not to bother—so I could keep ice on my hip for hours at a time. She got crutches. Why would I need crutches? It's just one hip! Sometimes my wife worries too much.

It turns out, I used all of it—the meds, the ice, *and* the crutches. And while the pain after the first surgery was fairly manageable, the procedure—an effort to restore the blood flow to my hip—was a failure. Time for the next step: a total hip replacement.

Statistically, about 94 percent of hip replacement surgeries go well and people have far less pain afterward than they did before.[4] But someone, I suppose, has to be in the unlucky 6 percent. It didn't take long for the doctor and me to conclude that my surgery hadn't gone well. He tried two more surgeries to fix things, but I continued to experience more pain. I got a second . . . and third . . . and fourth opinions, and each of them agreed that another surgery was necessary. I chose a doctor who specializes in revising hip replacements gone bad. He fixed one of the problems caused by the first replacement but, in the process, created other issues that haven't gone away. As a further complication from the last surgery, I got sick and stayed sick for months. It was a degree of misery I had never experienced.

Now in time, of course, I got better. My incisions healed. The X-rays looked good. I started to gain back some weight. I returned to work.

But I still hurt, far more than I had expected I would. The pain persisted, which made no sense to me. In large part, the problem presumably had been fixed. And I was very unhappy about it and not entirely shy about letting people know.

So I was referred to a different kind of doctor. The orthopedic surgeons had done what they could, so it was time to visit a specialist: a "pain management" doctor. Frankly, I didn't want to go, even though I was in pain, because I wasn't willing to concede that my pain was never going to go away. It felt like an admission of weakness, of failure. If I was a stronger person—which I thought I was, after being a Christian for most of my life—I shouldn't need someone to tell me how to manage my pain. I was embarrassed to tell my friends I had been referred to a pain management doctor.

But I didn't seem to have any other options, and I owed it to my wife and the people whose lives were impacted by my pain to try everything I could, so I made the appointment. My personal physician was fairly insistent upon it, as well. The first specialist I visited prescribed a medicine used to treat nerve pain. It turns out there are some people who have significant psychological reactions to those drugs. After getting "lost" in our shower and becoming so confused that I couldn't figure out how to turn off the water, my wife and I surmised that I just might be one of those people. A second drug caused a similar extreme result, so I stopped taking the drugs.

I then tried some other pain-management techniques, and if you've suffered from chronic pain, you've likely tried them too. There's TENS therapy—transcutaneous electrical nerve stimulation. Lidocaine patches. Exercises from a physical therapist. Steroid injections. Pain meds—hydrocodone, morphine, oxycodone. Ice became my best friend. I went to sleep with two ice packs on my back and two on my hip every night for months. I used ice packs while I drove and while I sat in my chair at work.

One of my emotional low points came with a visit to a pain-management specialist recommended to me by a friend. I went with high hopes that this doctor could help me. I brought my MRI results, my medical records, and a clear write-up of my story. But about halfway through the appointment, I noticed he wasn't interested in my records or my story He did recommend I buy and read a particular book, however, and he said I needed to take a six-week-long, eight-hours-a-day course on pain management. I would learn things like art therapy, he said. My wife cringed—she's seen me try to draw. But it was his diagnosis of my problem that jolted me. "Your karma has been disrupted. We need to address your karma."

I am told that this doctor has helped many people manage their pain, but I knew he wasn't going to help me. I am not an expert in Eastern religions, but I understand them well enough to know that karma is a Buddhist doctrine largely at odds with how I read the Bible. So I thanked him for his time, politely declined his invitation to take his class, and left.

Oh, and I went home to pout.

Looking back, I now realize why my experience with pain-management doctors was so disappointing. I really didn't want their help *managing* my pain; I wanted them to *eliminate* my pain. But that's not what they do. It's a hard truth—*sometimes the pain doesn't go away, no matter what.* And that's when you go to a pain-management doctor: when the pain persists even after the injury has healed and when medical science can't identify the cause of the pain.

CRAIG SELNESS

If you're in chronic pain, there's a great deal pain-management specialists can do to help you, assuming that you are realistic about what they can and can't do. They really can provide an invaluable service. Pain—as you know—is very personal, and a specialist of pain-management is better equipped than most general practitioners to help discover what works to get a grip on your particular pain. Ice has become a good friend to me, and myofascial massage continues to benefit me in tangible ways. But art therapy made me feel all the more helpless (in no world can what I do be called "art.") On the other hand, a friend of mine finds art therapy to be, well, therapeutic, while ice and massages just make her more miserable.

But I wanted to learn much more than how to manage my pain. I didn't like my pain. But, worse, *I didn't like me.* Yes, I did need to learn how to manage my *pain*, but far more importantly, I needed to learn how to manage my *life*.

Let me try to explain what I mean when I say that, because of my pain, I didn't like me. It's not that I became a constant complainer. It's not that I was mean to people (well, maybe I was, a little). It's not that I cursed God. But I had an overwhelming sense that, as a person and as a follower of Jesus, I was becoming smaller. Part of that is because my world, for a couple of years, in fact did become smaller. For a time, my world consisted of my recliner, which was basically the only place where I felt comfortable. As time went on, my world began to get bigger; today I can go most of the places I really want to. But while my world got bigger, I didn't. At least, I didn't *feel* I like I was getting bigger.

More specifically, here's what was—and to a degree, is— painful to me about me. I had always been a spiritually and

26

professionally ambitious person, someone who thrived on setting goals and being disciplined and pushing myself to get better. But as the physical pain lingered, I could feel those parts of me shriveling up. I was becoming apathetic about my spiritual life. The spiritual habits I had practiced for decades—Bible reading, memorizing verses, listening to Christian music, prayer, talking to people about my faith—interested me less and less. It's not that I was having doubts about my faith or that I was particularly angry with God. I just didn't want to do those things anymore.

And it wasn't just my spiritual life. I was becoming apathetic about life itself. Did you ever have a time when you couldn't do something you loved and part of how you coped with the frustration was to tell yourself that you didn't care, that you didn't really want to do that thing anyway? That's very much what I did, but I didn't stop there. I not only told myself I didn't care that I couldn't do some of the things I *used* to do; I told myself that I didn't care about many of the things *I could still do*.

And when you're in pain, it's a little easier to excuse your apathy and shallowness. Dealing with pain takes a fair bit of energy, so it's only natural (you tell yourself) that you have less grit and ambition for the rest of your life. And if someone challenges you and tells you that you are capable of doing more or of being better, you have a ready response: "You don't understand. You don't know what I'm going through." How can anyone argue with that? But it doesn't have to be that way.

Time for Some Good News

There is good news for us who live in pain, however; in the Bible it's called "the gospel." That word "gospel," as you might have read, means "good news," and the gospel of Jesus described in the Bible offers people in pain all the good news they need.

And, to clarify, I'm talking about good *news*, not good *advice*.

When we tell people about our issues with pain, most people want to offer us some good advice. Much of it is helpful, and some not so much. But even the best advice—write out your feelings, take this supplement, listen to this music, find a hobby—is of limited utility. Because often it's not so much that we don't know what to do or how we should act; *it's that we can't do it.* It feels like something in us is broken and there's nothing we can do to fix it, even if you tell us exactly what to do. And you can challenge us to "try harder" or to "give it some time," but it only makes us feel frustrated and a little bit ashamed, because we have tried harder and we have given it some time.

The Bible says this: "For the kingdom of God is not a matter of talk but of power" (1 Corinthians 4:20). The gospel is not simply good advice on how to manage our pain; the gospel is the good news that God can and will give us the power to manage our pain well. It's not merely good advice on how to manage your life; it's the ability to manage what seems unmanageable.

I'm at the age where I need reading glasses. My "near" vision used to be perfect, but now, especially in the mornings, I have great difficulty focusing my eyes on words and objects close to me. It does not help to "try harder." As you may well know from personal experience, "trying harder" does not bring focus to blurry letters. And there is no advice you can give me that will solve my problem. But when I pull out my reading glasses (three pairs for $9.99 at the local drugstore!), suddenly I can see. Before putting on my glasses, the text messages on my phone were largely illegible; afterward, I can read them without a problem.

The message of the gospel is not to "try harder." The message of the gospel is the good news that God can empower us to manage our pain with grace and dignity and hope and even joy. Good advice can't fix what pain has broken in our hearts and souls, but God can. He can enlarge the hearts our pain seemed to shrink. He may not take away the pain, but He can and will restore our souls. He can give us everything we need to live with our pain without our *being* pains too.

I mentioned that, in his letters, the Apostle Peter has quite a bit to say about pain and suffering. Near the end of his first letter to a church filled with folk like you and me, Peter offers us this piece of good news: "And the God of all grace, who called you to his eternal glory in Christ, after you have suffered a little while, will himself restore you and make you strong, firm and steadfast" (1 Peter 5:10).

The unpleasant truth is that sometimes the pain doesn't go away. But our lives? Here's the good news: by the grace of God, those can be restored.

The Greek word Peter uses for "restore" is *katartizo*. In some places in the New Testament, *katartizo* is translated in various Bible versions as "to mend" or "to repair," such as when fishermen would mend their damaged nets (Matthew 4:21). In other places, it's translated as "equip," "train," or "prepare"; in Ephesians 4:12, Paul explains that God gave pastors and teachers to the church to "equip his people for works of service." A bit more technically, *katartizo* is a combination of the root words "kata," which means "down," and "artios," which means to "properly adjust" something so that it works the way it was designed to work.[5]

I am not good at repair work. If something in our home breaks, my remedy is to throw it out and buy a new one. My wife and my son-in-law, Scott, don't throw things away. They seem to look forward to things breaking just so they can find creative ways to repair or adjust them. (They're a little like the TV character "MacGyver.") For example, the reclining mechanism in my favorite chair broke. I wanted to haul the chair to the curb and get a new one. (I think we can agree that there is no point to a recliner that doesn't recline.) My wife would have none of it; she contended that we could fix it. So we ordered the replacement part and went to work once it arrived. I had an important role: I held the flashlight. Brenda twisted some things, taped some things (duct tape to the rescue), adjusted some things, and voilà! My chair reclines again. Now, if you were to look underneath the chair, you would notice that it does not look "as good as new." Nor does it function as smoothly as it did before it broke. But it works; it reclines like it was designed to do. My wife was able to *katartizo* my chair.

There is a sense in which chronic pain breaks some of who we are on the inside. It can sap us of our energy, our ambition, and our will. It can make it feel impossible to function normally. But God can restore us. He can mend us; He can equip us; He can adjust our hearts and souls so they once again work the way God designed them to work.

That's the good news. And because of it, we can manage our pain without being pains, to others or to ourselves.

So let's discover just how this good news really works.

"When I don't know what to think:
Tracking truth we can trust."

CHAPTER THREE

O ver the last few years, my wife has often asked me a particular question. She would see that I was having a hard time, that I was struggling in one way or another with my pain, and she would say: "So what are you telling yourself?" At first, I didn't like it when she asked me that. No, that's not true; I *never* like it when she asks me that. Yes, she's asking a question, but she's also making a statement, and I don't really want to hear it. I don't want to hear that the reason I'm struggling might well have more to do with what I'm thinking than what's going on with my sensory neurons. Now, she isn't suggesting—nor am I—that the pain is "all in my head." But she is reminding me that one key to living with pain without becoming one is the conversation I'm having with myself.

There's nothing odd about talking to yourself; we all do it. We even see it in the Bible. The psalmist was remarkably candid about what he was telling himself during a rough patch in his life: "Why, my soul, are you downcast? Why so disturbed within me? Put your hope in God, for I will yet praise him, my Savior and my God" (Psalm 42:5). The psalmist was depressed and he wasn't sure why, so he had a talk with himself: "What's the problem? Why are you sad?" And then he did the healthy thing—he gave himself a pep talk: "Trust God. He'll help you handle whatever is dragging you down."

When my wife asks me, "So what are you telling yourself?" my first response to her is usually the standard male answer to any such question: "Nothing." Actually, that response is partially correct—I'm not conscious of the fact that I'm telling myself anything. But Brenda will gently (her word, not mine) push me to think a little harder about my answer, and after a few moments of reflection, here's what I realize I'm telling myself:

"I'm never going to get better."

"This isn't fair."

"I don't think I can do this much longer."

"Nobody really understands how this feels."

"There is no point to this."

"There has to be something I can do to make this better, but I have no idea what it is."

Perhaps you've told yourself something similar ("I give up." "Why doesn't someone help me?" "Being a 'good sport' about all this isn't helping me, so maybe I'll just do what I feel like doing for a while"). And I don't blame you. I think those are very natural and reasonable thoughts for a person in chronic pain to have. In fact, there's likely a fair bit of truth in many of those statements. For example, while your symptoms will probably improve, you may never get completely well again, so in that sense, you may never get better. And fair? No, most of the time, what you're going through isn't fair. But—and you already know this—those aren't particularly helpful, healing, or productive thoughts to tell yourself. I

knew that even before my wife helped me say it out loud. I knew
that what I was telling myself was making me feel more hopeless,
more depressed, and more resentful. I knew those thoughts weren't
helping me cope with my pain, and they weren't helping me be the
person I wanted to be.

But this was the problem: *I didn't know what to think.*

Here's what I mean. I knew that it would likely be helpful
for me to think positive thoughts; to tell myself, "You're going to
get better"; to sing with Little Orphan Annie, "The sun will come
out tomorrow"; to feed my mind with happy or healing ideas and
images. . . . But the skeptical side of me would pull me up short.
That part of me would not allow me to tell myself thoughts I was
not convinced were *true.*

For example, if you've been to a pain-management specialist
or if you've read up on pain-management techniques, you've likely
learned that you can manage the intensity of your pain with your
thoughts. One technique, for example, is called "mental anesthe-
sia." In this technique, as I have had it explained to me, you use
the power of your mind to imagine injecting a numbing anesthetic
into the painful area or applying an ice pack to the place of pain.
I have been told by some people that this is quite helpful. Yet my
mind stubbornly resists such techniques, because the voice in my
head keeps telling me, "But it's not true."

It may not be helpful to tell myself, "This isn't fair." Actually,
there's no "may" about it—it's not helpful. But, I reasoned, at least
that's true—isn't it? Yes, fairness is a tricky concept. Who am I
to know what is ultimately *fair* about my life versus the life of
any other human being? And yet in some limited fashion, it seems
reasonable for me to conclude that it is *not* fair that 94 percent of

people who had my surgeries have so much less pain than me. And I imagine that, in large measure, what has happened to you simply isn't fair either.

So I'll say it again—I didn't know what to think.

JOB DIDN'T KNOW WHAT TO THINK

Job didn't know what to think. No, I'm not in *any* way comparing myself to Job. He endured more pain than a person should be asked to suffer. And when he said to himself and to his friends, "This isn't fair," he was telling the whole truth. God Himself exonerated Job when God said this about Job to Satan: "Have you considered my servant Job? There is no one on earth like him; he is blameless and upright, a man who fears God and shuns evil" (Job 1:8). So Job's protestations of innocence to his friends were completely valid; his claim that his suffering was undeserved was objectively true.

So, then, what is Job to think? He's not sure. His suffering makes no sense. So Job spends a fair bit of time talking to himself. Sometimes Job talks to his friends, Eliphaz, Bildad, Zophar, and Elihu. And other times Job talks to God. But, in essence, much of what Job says, he says to himself. And what does he tell himself?

I'm never going to get better.
    —"My eyes will never see happiness again" (Job 7:7);
    "my gnawing pains never rest" (Job 30:17).

This isn't fair.
    —"As surely as God lives, who has denied me
    justice . . ." (Job 27:2).

I don't think I can do this much longer.

—"What I feared has come upon me; what I dreaded has happened to me. I have no peace, no quietness; I have no rest, but only turmoil" (Job 3:25–26).

Nobody really understands how this feels.

—"He has alienated my family from me; my acquaintances are completely estranged from me. My relatives have gone away; my closest friends have forgotten me" (Job 19:13–14).

There is no point to this.

—"I despise my life; I would not live forever. Let me alone; my days have no meaning" (Job 7:16).

There has to be something I can do to make this better, but I have no idea what it is.

—"When I think my bed will comfort me and my couch will ease my complaint, even then you frighten me with dreams and terrify me with visions, so that I prefer strangling and death, rather than this body of mine" (Job 7:13–15).

In large part Job said to himself many of the same things we tell ourselves when we're in pain. And in large part, the things he said to himself were as helpful as the things we say to ourselves, which is to say . . . not very helpful at all.

Now to Job's credit, he does tell himself some hopeful things. As the saying goes, "Never doubt in the dark what you've learned in the light," and even in his pain Job reminds himself of some truths he'd come to believe in his better days: "I know that my redeemer lives, and that in the end he will stand on the earth. And after my skin has been destroyed, yet in my flesh I will see God; I myself will see him with my own eyes—I, and not another" (Job 19:25–27). Job interspersed his dark and depressing thoughts with hopeful thoughts. And most of the time, so do we. Even those with the most melancholy bent allow themselves a few moments of happy, healing, and hopeful meditations.

But then the next setback comes (the pain ratchets up, a friend doesn't show, the doctor has bad news . . .), and so do our darker thoughts. We need help. We need someone to teach us how to think. God did just that for Job. He didn't do it the way Job hoped He would, though. He didn't come to Job and say, "Job, let Me tell you why this is happening to you. Let Me explain to you the cause of your curse and the point of your pain." That's what Job wanted, what he had asked for, and precisely what God did *not* do. Instead, God asked Job a long series of questions, none of which Job could possibly answer. And in asking Job those questions, God taught Job what to think, which is this: *Sometimes God only knows, and because He loves me, that's all I need to know.*

Now here's the really interesting thing about the book of Job. God never explains to Job why he's suffering. But He does explain it to us. God told Job all Job needed to know, which was, "I've got this, and I love you, so trust Me." But God tells *us* the backstory. God takes us behind the scenes to show us far more about what was going on than Job ever knew. And while we'll explore a bit later some of the truth God reveals to us in the book of Job, here's the bigger point: *God wants us to know how to think.*

That's not to say God offers to provide us with an exhaustive and complete explanation of our suffering and pain; He doesn't. But here is the good news—*God does offer to show us everything we need to know in order to live with pain without becoming one.* He offers to tell us the truth we need to know, and He offers to give us the grace that restores our souls.

GOD CHANGES OUR LIVES BY CHANGING OUR MINDS

When you're living in pain, whether it's physical or emotional pain, you just want to make a change, somehow. You want to change the past—the accident, the mistake, the surgery, the heartbreak, the event that has led you to *this*, whatever *this* is. You want to change whatever it is that is keeping you stuck in your misery. Something has to change, even if you don't quite know what.

I'm a bit embarrassed to tell you this, but sometimes I like watching those made-for-TV movies that always have a "happily-ever-after" ending on the Hallmark Channel. Oh, I watch my share of action flicks and thrillers, as well, but once in a while I really appreciate watching a story about people whose lives turn out just peachy.

One night my wife and I sat down to watch one of those movies called *Remember Sunday* starring Zachary Levi, who had previously been the star of a silly but fun spy show called *Chuck*. Levi played a character on *Remember Sunday* named Gus, a brilliant scientist who had suffered a brain aneurysm that left him with a severe short-term-memory issue. His long-term memory was intact, but he was unable to remember anything that had happened the day before. His apartment is filled with Post-it notes that serve as his short-term memory to remind him what happened and who he met the previous day. But it's a painfully hard way to live and a particularly difficult way to develop any new relationships.

One day his sister takes Gus to his regular doctor. He's hoping for some good news; he's hoping to hear that he's getting better, that someday his short-term memory will be restored. But the doctor tells him that there is no such hope; this, sadly, is as good as it gets.

Up until this point in the story, Gus has been positive and strong; he has carried himself with dignity and grace. But when the doctor tells him that he'll never get better, Gus begins to sob uncontrollably. He finally composes himself enough to explain his tears: "I can't do this anymore. I can't live like this."

My wife, I could tell, was trying not to look at me, and for good reason. Because as soon as she did, I began to sob too. Gus had said exactly what I had been feeling for some time. I knew I wasn't supposed to feel that way. After all, I was the pastor of a church. The very next morning, I would be standing in front of our church, doing my best to communicate a message of hope and faith and joy. Yet a part of me was very much afraid that I just couldn't handle my life for one more day. I desperately needed something to change, and at that moment there seemed to be little hope that I or anyone else could do anything to change the things that were making me so miserable.

Ever been there? Ever hit a wall emotionally, ever feel like you just didn't have it in you to keep hoping and trying? Do you remember where you were and what you were thinking when life gave you a punch in the gut?

So then here's the question. How does the good news of the gospel work when you can't change your circumstances? It works by changing you. And this is where it begins: *God changes our lives by changing our minds.* He changes our attitudes and even our emotions by changing how we think and what we believe. And the result is, while He may not restore our health or our circumstances, He most certainly will restore what needs it most—our souls.

David, the shepherd boy who became the second king of Israel, put it like this in the most famous of all psalms: "The LORD is my shepherd, I shall not be in want. He makes me lie down in green pastures, he leads me beside quiet waters, he restores my soul" (Psalm 23:1–3 NIV84). Peter, remembered for denying his Lord three times before experiencing reconciliation with Jesus and the restoration of his soul, discovered that God Himself restores us and make us strong (1 Peter 5:10).

And let's remember an important distinction—the gospel is not good advice on how to restore your soul or on how to make your life better. The gospel is good news, the good news that the God of all grace Himself will restore our souls. He is the one who changes us, who makes us well, who heals our brokenness. And that process of transformation begins with our minds: "Do not conform any longer to the pattern of this world, but be transformed by the renewing of your mind" (Romans 12:2 NIV84). God changes our lives by changing how we think.

So what are we supposed to think? When it comes to pain and grief and loss and misery and frustration and despair, what are we supposed to think?

When you read the New Testament letters of Paul, you'll

notice that he talks quite a lot about how to think. In Romans 8, for example, a chapter in which Paul's focus is to explain how to change your life and how to be free of all the urges and impulses that drag us down, Paul says this: "Those who live according to the sinful nature have their minds set on what that nature desires; but those who live in accordance with the Spirit have their minds set on what the Spirit desires" (Romans 8:5 NIV84). Clearly our "mind-set" is critical to changing who we are so that we are able to live with pain without becoming one. But we could really use some precision; what *specifically* are we supposed to think about?

And Paul obliges us. It's a great summary statement of what God wants us to think, and it's found in Paul's letter to the Philippians. Paul is writing this from an underground prison cell in Rome, unsure whether he'll ever get out. We're actually not sure how long it was after this that Paul was martyred. And yet Philippians is a book that drips with joy. How could Paul be joyful when his circumstances were, quite frankly, miserable? What was Paul supposed to think? He tells us: "Finally, brothers and sisters, whatever is true, whatever is noble, whatever is right, whatever is pure, whatever is lovely, whatever is admirable—if anything is excellent or praiseworthy—think about such things" (Philippians 4:8).

Notice what's first on Paul's list of things to think about: *whatever is true.* The key to life transformation and soul restoration is truth. So when it comes to our pain, what's the truth? The Bible has a great deal to say about that. Of course, the Bible doesn't tell us everything we'd like to know about pain, particularly about our own pain. *But while the Bible doesn't tell us everything, everything it tells us is true.*

We'll start with some hard truth, the truth about the pain that's our own fault. As you can imagine, the news about this kind of pain is not all good. But there is still good news to be had, and it comes down to one familiar yet still amazing truth—the truth the Bible calls "grace."

"When it's my own fault: Managing self-inflicted pain."

CHAPTER FOUR

So here's the first truth God wants us to understand about pain: sometimes our pain is our own fault. That doesn't make it hurt any less, of course. In some ways, that just makes the whole experience all the worse, because in addition to the pain, there's shame and guilt and embarrassment and regret mixed into the equation.

The first sports biography I ever read was one of Mickey Mantle, the celebrated outfielder for the New York Yankees; I'd had a chance to watch him play against my beloved Minnesota Twins in the 1960s. Some time ago, I was watching a replay of an interview of the legend, who died in 1995.[1] In that interview, Mantle—who, as it happened, didn't have long to live—was taking a look back on his life. The interviewer asked Mantle how he would sum up his life and career. I expected him to answer about his place in baseball history . . . his home runs, batting titles, MVP trophies, World Series rings, and all the success he'd enjoyed in life. But he didn't.

Instead, in an incredibly candid moment, Mantle—obviously speaking from a place of great pain—began to describe his regrets. He said he regretted that he had never become the player he had the ability to be because of his abuse of alcohol.. He regretted that because of his selfishness, he had never seen any of his four sons born. He regretted that he never gave any attention or affection to his son Billy in part because Billy was mentally and physically disabled. He regretted his rudeness to his friends and to his fans who just wanted to know him better. He regretted much of what he had done and who he had become.

Mantle managed to reverse things a bit in the last couple of years of his life. He went to rehab, gave up drinking, and did his best to warn people of the dangers of the self-destructive lifestyle he'd had. But the damage had been done, and Mantle was very honest about the fact that his pain, and the pain he had caused those around him, was quite his own fault.

The Bible has a great deal to say about the messes we make. And I know—we don't really want to hear about it. It's not fun to talk about those times when our pain is self-inflicted, when we hurt because, well, let's just say it—because we sinned.

But that's only part of the message, and it is *not* the last word on the matter. Let me be sure to headline the good news: *when it comes to the messes of our own making, grace gets the last word.* As evidence, the very last verse of the Bible is a word of grace: "The grace of the Lord Jesus be with God's people. Amen" (Revelation 22:21).

Zeke Pike was an All-American high-school quarterback in Kentucky who enrolled at Auburn on a full scholarship. He was being touted as the next Cam Newton; everything was going his way. Then his life went off the rails, and he readily admits that it was his own fault. He lost his scholarship when he was arrested on drug charges. He got hooked on Xanax, a sedative for the treatment of anxiety. Pike was ashamed that he had thrown away his athletic career, and his drug habit caused a significant rift with his family. Pike was literally on his way to committing suicide when he was arrested for driving under the influence of drugs.

But there's more to Zeke Pike's story than wasted potential and addiction. Like my grandfather, Pike's grandfather was a Baptist minister, and while in prison, Pike used his time to reconnect with the God he'd first discovered in his youth. In December 2016, just a month out of prison, Pike founded an organization called Number8 Ministries, a name he chose to represent new beginnings. He has reconciled with his family and devoted himself to sharing his story of pain and redemption. There will certainly be much more to the story of Zeke Pike, but at this moment, his story is surely a testament to God's amazing grace.[2]

THE CURSE AND OUR PAIN

But before we fully appreciate the good news of grace, we need to understand just what the bad news is. Or let me say it like this: to understand the big picture about living with the pain that's our own fault, we need to understand something about curses.

One of the best-known curses of recent times is one Chicago Cubs fans blamed for their team's extended World Series drought . . . the Curse of the Billy Goat. The Cubs were between World Series titles from 1908 through 2016, and their fans in part blamed a curse based on an odd event that took place when the Cubs played the Detroit Tigers in the 1945 World Series. Tavern owner William Sianis bought a ticket to Game 4 of the series for his pet billy goat, Murphy, but they were denied entrance to the game because of the goat's unpleasant smell. As they walked away from Wrigley Field, Sianis pronounced a curse: "You are going to lose this World Series, and you're never going to win another World Series again!"[3] Cubs fans everywhere took great joy in seeing the end of that curse when their much-loved team beat the Cleveland Indians in seven games in the 2016 World Series.

In many ways, the story of our pain is wrapped up in the story of a curse—a curse described in the very first book of the Bible, the book of Genesis. God creates Adam and Eve, Genesis tells us, and places them in a garden. God gives them a command—a rather simple command, actually—they could eat the fruit of any tree in the garden except for the fruit of one particular tree. You remember what happens: Adam and Eve exercise their free will; they make the choice to disobey God. And God then does what He warned He would do—*He pronounces a curse*. Here's the text from Genesis:

> To the woman he said, "I will make your pains in child-bearing very severe; with painful labor you will give birth to children. Your desire will be for your husband, and he will rule over you."
>
> To Adam he said, "Because you listened to your wife and ate fruit from the tree about which I commanded you, 'You must not eat from it,' "Cursed is the ground because of you; through painful toil you will eat food from it all the days of your life. . . . For dust you are and to dust you will return" (vv. 3:16–19).

But here's the more obvious point, though not a pleasant one— *the curse is our own fault*. Why are you and I in pain? This is *part* of the answer, something God wants us to know. Humankind messed up right from the beginning, and so, in the larger sense, we have no one to blame but ourselves. To a certain degree, the Bible teaches, much of what is wrong in our world is wrong because of the Fall of mankind. Much of the pain we suffer is because of the curse. Isaiah puts it this way: "Therefore a curse consumes the earth; its people must bear their guilt" (Isaiah 24:6).

It would be nice if there was a book in the Bible—or even just one chapter—in which God explained to us in precise detail why pain and suffering are such a big part of our world. There isn't, of course. The Bible wasn't written like a textbook that covers distinct topics in different chapters; it's a collection of stories and songs and letters written to real people who lived many hundreds of years ago. But as we observed earlier, God wants us to know how to think about pain, and there are a number of critical passages where the writers of the Bible get right to the point. Once such passage is in Romans 8:20–22, where we read this: "For the creation was subjected to frustration, not by its own choice, but by the will of the one who subjected it, in hope that the creation itself will be liberated from its bondage to decay and brought into the glorious freedom of the children of God. We know that the whole creation has been groaning as in the pains of childbirth right up to the present time" (NIV84).

Yes, that's a bit of a mouthful. But when we read carefully, it's not at all hard to see the echoes of Genesis 3 and the curse in those verses—"the whole creation has been groaning as in the pains of childbirth." One reason we experience pain is because creation is broken and, according to the Bible, humankind broke it when Adam and Eve sinned. One day the curse will be reversed, the Bible assures us (Revelation 22:3), but until that day we humans live with the consequences of an act of free will.

In some ways it's like a whole bunch of dominoes falling. The world record for the number of dominoes knocked over by tipping just the first domino is . . . 4,491,863, set in 2009 in the Netherlands on "Domino Day."[4] The sin of Adam and Eve was, in a way, the knocking over of the first domino, and thousands of years later the dominoes are still falling. There is pain and brokenness and heartache in our world because of the curse, and the unhappy truth is that we as mankind have no one to blame but ourselves.

I know. I want to argue the point myself: "The Fall of mankind isn't my fault. I didn't eat the apple; Adam and Eve did. It's their fault; you can't hang that on me." Two quick thoughts about that. Yes, Adam and Eve sinned first, but we've all sinned. None of us are off the hook. Also, let me acknowledge something: we don't fully understand how the "the creation was subjected to frustration" because of the Fall of Adam and Eve. But we don't need to. If we really needed to fully comprehend it before we could learn how to live with pain, I'm confident God would have given us a fuller explanation. As we've said before, *the Bible doesn't tell us everything, but everything it tells us is true.* And the truth is that in one way, the pain we experience in this world is because we as human beings have messed up morally. In the age to come, there will be no more pain (Revelation 21:4). But in the here and now, in this fallen world, pain is never far away.

GOD'S GRACIOUS DISCIPLINE

So that's some of the big picture about why there's pain in our lives, in all our lives. But let's bring it back to you and me. Is it possible that our pain is in some way our own fault, even if we're not aware that we specifically did anything wrong?

If someone drives drunk and crashes their car, well, sure, it's their own fault. It's not the last word for that person, though; as we will see again and again, anyone who suffers self-inflicted pain has the chance to make grace be the last word of their story. But what about, for example, the person who suffers from miserable back pain and did nothing to cause it? What does any of this have to do with us?

Have you ever had a well-meaning person suggest that God purposely caused your pain as a way of disciplining you? I have, and my wife has, and our first reaction was not . . . receptive. Brenda, in addition to experiencing the pain of giving birth, has had two other very painful episodes in her life. About twenty years ago, an elderly man in a large pickup truck ran a red light and T-boned Brenda's car right after she dropped off our youngest at preschool. To this day, Brenda has memory loss caused by the accident, and for the better part of three years she had terrible migraines and other physical pain that made her life extremely challenging.

A few years later Brenda developed back pain unlike anything I'd ever seen. Before one doctor's appointment, the pain was so severe that she couldn't manage to stand up, and when I tried to carry her, the pain was even worse. But she was determined to see the doctor, so she did a combat crawl from the parking lot to the doctor's office (and I was quite sure that everyone watching thought I was the worst husband in the world). After a few injections, disc surgery, and hours of physical therapy, her back is now fine. But the misery lasted for years.

And during her time of misery, one of the members of our church came to visit us and talk to Brenda about "a concern on her heart." She wondered what Brenda might have done to cause God to bring this pain into her life. She wondered if God had revealed to Brenda why it was that He was disciplining her with this pain.

She actually said it with kindness, sincerity, and the best of intentions. But I'll be honest, we didn't think it was her place to say it. It certainly wasn't the *time* to say it. Someone said something similar to me when I was at my worst, and again, at the time it was not a particularly helpful thing to say. And yet—though it pains me a bit to admit it—those folks had a point, a point that has the potential for helping me live with my pain without becoming one. Here's what I mean.

According to the Bible, there is a certain kind of pain God *intentionally* brings into our lives as a means of disciplining us, as a way of correcting us when we veer off course morally. Job 5:17 says this: "Blessed is the one whom God corrects; so do not despise the discipline of the Almighty." In the last book of the Bible, Jesus says this to the church at Laodicea: "Those whom I love I rebuke and discipline. So be earnest, and repent" (Revelation 3:19 NIV84). Did you ever get disciplined as a kid? I have to imagine that all of us were; I certainly was. It wasn't fun; we didn't like it. But we probably deserved it. And if it was done properly, if it was received properly, it made us better people.

Sometimes I'll hear people say that God never causes pain, that He is too loving and gracious to ever purposely bring pain into our lives. But the Bible is quite clear about this—that's just not true. The truth is that God is too loving and gracious to *not* bring pain into our lives. But the Bible is loud and clear about God's intentions. The purpose of God's discipline is not to punish us, but to correct us and to shape us into the people we want to be.

This, by the way, is a critically important distinction to keep in mind. When God brings pain into the lives of His followers, He's not doing it to punish us. It's tempting to think that's what's happening; it's a common reaction. But the gospel message could not be clearer—*Jesus already took the punishment for our sins.*

The author of Hebrews reminds his readers that "Christ was sacrificed once to take away the sins of many . . ." and that "by one sacrifice he has made perfect forever those who are being made holy" (Hebrews 9:28; 10:14). Jesus paid for our sins on the cross. The forgiveness of our sins is made possible by Jesus's suffering and death, *not by our pain.* And that's a message we all need to be reminded of, especially when life is hard. You lost your job? You lost your wife? You're sick and you don't know if you're going to get well? Here's the truth: these things aren't happening to you because God is punishing you. Your sin is forgiven. The price has already been paid.

But the rest of the story is this—*sometimes God brings pain into our lives not to punish us but to get us back on track morally.* Here is the most complete treatment of this topic in the Bible:

Endure hardship as discipline; God is treating you as his children. For what children are not disciplined by their father? If you are not disciplined—and everyone undergoes discipline—then you are not legitimate, not true sons and daughters at all. Moreover, we have all had human fathers who disciplined us and we respected them for it. How much more should we submit to the Father of spirits and live! They disciplined us for a little while as they thought best; but God disciplines us for our good, in order that we may share in his holiness. No discipline seems pleasant at the time, but painful. Later on, however, it produces a harvest of righteousness and peace for those who have been trained by it. (Hebrews 12:7–11)

My dad served as a marine in WWII, and there were times growing up when I regretted that marine background. I came to value the discipline my dad built into my life; it served me well in sports and in school. But at the time, it was painful. We had fifty-three trees on our property in the suburbs of the Twin Cities, and around each tree was a well. One of my jobs as a youngster was to trim those tree wells a few times a year to make sure they were perfect circles and no weeds or grass invaded their space. Initially I did not think that having perfectly circular tree wells was a high priority in my life, especially when my friends were out playing ball and riding bikes. But my dad corrected my misunderstanding; he taught me that a job worth doing was worth doing as well as one could.

The Hall of Fame ex-coach of the Dallas Cowboys, the late Tom Landry once said, "The job of a coach is to make men do what they do not want to do, in order that they can be what they've always wanted to be." Or, again, as Jesus Himself said it, "Those whom I love I rebuke and discipline" (Revelation 3:19). So the question then becomes, "How do I live with it?"

In part, this is an easy answer, and in part it's actually pretty hard. The easy answer is this—repent. That's how Jesus told us to respond when He rebukes and disciplines us, by repenting. Part of repenting is to grieve over our wrongdoing, to lament our moral lameness. But primarily, to repent is to change direction and get back on the right path. And that's all well and good if it's clear you've done something for which you need to repent. If you steal the cash from your church's weekly offerings to help pay for your addiction to prescription pain medication and God brings additional hardship into your life, it's not difficult to discern the first step you need to take—repenting and making things right—because in the long run, your character matters far more than your comfort.

OUR PAIN: PART OF GOD'S DISCIPLINE?

But what if you haven't done anything blatantly wrong? Is it possible that God is still bringing pain into your life to correct something that you've missed? *How do you know when God is disciplining you?*

I've asked myself that many times over the last few years. I'm not saying that my sin was the direct cause of my hip problems and all the issues that came with five surgeries. It's not like my hip went bad because I abused drugs or ate an ungodly number of Arby's sandwiches (which I have). But I have asked myself, and I asked God, "Is this the hand of God to correct something in my life that's out of line? Am I missing something God is trying to help me see?"

We all learned about blind spots in driver's education. The novice driver mistakenly believes that he can see everything behind and next to him by looking in his mirrors. But he soon learns that unless he turns his head, there will be blind spots in his vision that could cause him great harm. There are times in our lives when everything looks quite right . . . until God does something, often something painful, to cause us to turn our head and see that flaw to which we had been blind. And that's what my wife's friend and my friend were asking about when they asked us whether God might have caused our pain to teach us a lesson; they were wondering if perhaps God might have been trying to get us to take a look at our blind spots.

Now here's something I've learned about this process over the years. I've learned that I am notoriously bad in discerning on my own whether God is, in fact, disciplining me. *This is where we really need each other in the Body of Christ.* We need to be able to go to people who know and love us, who are in touch with God, and ask them, "Do you see anything in my life that God might need to correct in me? Do you think it's possible that this particular pain might be the discipline of the Father?"

And even if most of the time the answer you settle on is, "No, I don't think this is the discipline of the Lord," it's still a healthy process to go through. It's still good for us to regularly check our hearts, our attitudes, and our actions to evaluate how closely we're following God's lead in our lives. Sometimes God brings pain into our lives to correct us because we've gotten off track morally and spiritually, and when He does, we need to handle it not by whining or complaining, but by taking the time to honestly assess whether we have a blind spot that needs our attention.

GOD'S OFFERING FOR
SELF-INFLICTED PAIN: GRACE

But the last word comes from the last verse of the Bible—*grace.* The good news for all of us is that God offers us grace when our pain is self-inflicted.

One of the places I have learned the most about this is from sitting in on the recovery meetings often held at our church. I've heard some very courageous folk stand up in front of the group and admit, "I have suffered a great deal and, frankly, it's been my fault. It's my fault for drinking more than I should and for driving when I've been drinking. No one made me drink, no one made me do drugs, no one made me gamble—it was my choice. I ended up in jail, I alienated my wife and family, and I lost my job. But the fact is that I did it to myself. And I have to live with the consequences of what I did."

But those same people went on to make something very clear—*there is life after self-inflicted pain.* That's good news, because every one of us has made more than our share of messes. We have caused pain to ourselves, and we have caused pain to those around us. And we have the scars to show it.

Have you seen the "Dog shaming" calendar? It's a picture a day of different dogs who have committed a variety of shameful acts, causing their owners to place signs around their necks describing the deeds. For example, one German shepherd wears a sign that says, "I jump up on the counter and eat pizza." A small mixed-breed dog wrapped in a phone line wears a sign that says, "I broke the Internet." Another dog sits on a ripped-apart couch and wears a sign that says, "I'm the reason Mommy and Daddy can't have nice things."

And it makes me think . . . what sign should I be wearing? Because, like all of us, I have acted badly and I have caused pain, and there are times when I feel like just hanging my head in shame.

But shame and regret and heartache and pain are not the end— grace has the last word. It is never too late to turn and run to our heavenly Father. None of us has fallen too far to be loved and accepted by the God who sent His Son to die so that our lives might be redeemed and remade. When our pain is our own fault, when our suffering is self-inflicted, we still have this option—to turn to the Father and receive His grace.

Kurt is one of my closest friends, though we could not be more different. Kurt had a pretty rough upbringing, which he parlayed into a life of drinking, drugs, and crime. As Kurt tells it, he was the reason people like me put alarms on our suburban homes and stay off the roads late at night. He was the guy we would point out to our kids and say, "That's what alcohol does to a person; that's what happens if you don't stay in school." Kurt doesn't have any training as a public speaker, but when he tells his story, the audience is spellbound; he's just done so many crazy things that we can't quite believe he's still alive (including jumping out of a car traveling 65 mph).

Eventually Kurt's poor choices caught up to him and he served his time. He got involved in AA and turned his life around. When I met Kurt, he had been sober for six or seven years but was still in the process of figuring out what life had for him. What I admired about Kurt right from the beginning was that he never blamed his upbringing or his genetics for the life he lived. He never claimed to have been a victim. He readily owned up to the fact that the mess he had made of his life was of his own making.

But while Kurt had come to believe in a "Higher Power" before coming to our church, he wasn't quite sure who that was or what that meant. I remember visiting Kurt at his house and seeing a shelf full of Bibles. When he saw me looking at them, he explained: "My family and friends keep giving me Bibles, thinking that's what I need. But I haven't read any of them; they don't make a lot of sense to me." Kurt was a willing student, though; he came to church every Sunday, got involved in small-group Bible studies, and started reading the Bible himself. And in time, Kurt chose to turn control of his life over to Jesus, and he demonstrated that commitment by choosing to get baptized.

In the last twenty years, Kurt has been influential in helping hundreds of struggling people turn their lives around. He leads a variety of AA meetings; he's sponsored scores of recovering addicts; he regularly visits the local jails. He is the poster child of a life redeemed. There was a time when Kurt was nothing but a pain to his family, his friends, to much of our community, and most of all, to himself. And now he is the first person you would call if you needed help. The pain Kurt experienced in life—and there has been quite a lot—was almost all self-inflicted. But for Kurt, shame and regret and pain are not the end. The last word is grace.

WHEN YOU'RE THE VICTIM

But wait—what about the victim? What about the pain of the person who suffers through no fault of their own? Here's the truth—when someone causes us pain, we want very much to become a pain to them. Tempting as that might be, there is a better way, a healthier way, to handle our unjust hurts. That's next.

"When I'm the victim: Managing unjust hurts."

CHAPTER FIVE

——————

Finding a movie that everyone in the family enjoys watching can be a challenge. Stereotypically, men like to watch action flicks and women like to watch romantic comedies—and that's largely true in our family as well. But there are two types of movies Brenda and I tend to agree on. For one thing, we tend to prefer true stories over pure fiction. Secondly, we both like a movie where the bad guy gets what's coming to him. Of course, we can't watch those movies with our kids; we've always taught them that it's wrong to "get even," so we don't really want them hearing us cheer for Liam Neeson, Matt Damon, or Jennifer Lopez to take their revenge on the fictional villain.

Now you may be thinking, "This might not be the kind of pastor I want to meet in a dark alley." So let me reassure you, we know it's wrong to take justice into our own hands. We know it's wrong under our legal system, and we know it's wrong as Christians. And I'm sure you know it's wrong too. But let me ask you this: have you ever been a victim . . . treated unjustly . . . or suffered at the hands of another person, and thought to yourself, "That's enough. I'm not going to take this anymore"?

In the last chapter I addressed the kind of pain we sometimes cause ourselves—self-inflicted pain. In this chapter, my focus is on what God wants us to know about how to handle unjust hurts— how to manage the pain that has been thrust upon us through no fault of our own.

In both situations, there are actually two different kinds of pain involved. For example, when your pain is your own fault, you experience both *physical pain* as well as the *shame* of having messed up. I have a friend who crashed his car into a light pole because he was under the influence of alcohol. He knew better than to drive after drinking, but he did it anyway. He happened to be a worship leader in his church. And as a result of that event, he suffered in two ways—physical pain from the accident and the shame of having let his family and his church down. I am glad to say that he responded to that painful event by doing everything right. He took ownership of his problem, he got into recovery, and he gave up drinking alcohol and replaced it by drinking deeply from the grace of God.

Like self-inflicted injuries, the hurts we suffer at the hands of others also cause two kinds of pain. First, there is the physical *and* emotional pain we suffer from the wrong done to us. If someone hits us for no good reason, for example, we hurt; if someone betrays us unjustly, we suffer. But there's another kind of pain we experience as well: *bitterness.* And I would imagine you know exactly what I'm talking about. Bitterness is a misery all its own.

Jerry is one of the first friends I made when I moved to California in 1979, and we are close to this day. Jerry's pain is different from mine; mine is mostly physical, and Jerry's is the pain of betrayal and loss. No one, I suppose, is entirely blameless when a marriage ends, but it's hard to see how his wife's affair was Jerry's fault. She then moved to another state and took their two young children with her, refusing to let Jerry have any contact with them. And while Jerry has managed his pain well all these years, it's always there in one way or another. Sometimes there's the temptation to be bitter. Other times it's a lingering sadness that hangs over every minute of every day. As Jerry puts it, it's like he's always standing under a large tree. He can see the sunshine, but he can never quite get out of the shade.

Does the Bible have anything to say to those who suffer from unjust hurts? Our goal is to discover how to live with pain without becoming one, but let's be honest—*when someone has caused us pain, we very much want to become a pain to them.* We want to turn the tables; we want revenge. But is that the right response? Silly question. We know it's not. But what we need to understand and believe is that it's not a *healthy* response, nor is it a *helpful* response. So what does the Bible have to say about how to handle unjust hurts in a healthy way for us and in a way that would make our God proud?

It turns out that the Bible has quite a lot to say about handling unjust hurts. And that makes sense when we think about it. After all, the One we follow—Jesus, the Christ—was a completely innocent man and yet suffered horrific pain at the hands of evil men. So we would expect the Bible to talk about that, and of course it does.

FORGIVENESS IS THE BEST OPTION

If you've heard or read any of the teachings of Jesus, you already know what I'm going to say: when you're suffering from an unjust hurt, the best option is forgiveness. But here's the hard reality:

it sure doesn't feel like the best option. In fact, it feels like a very bad option, like something you do if you're too weak to do anything else. Yes, we know Jesus was very clear about this, that He taught us in the Lord's Prayer to forgive as we've been forgiven (Matthew 6:14–15). But it just doesn't feel right; it doesn't feel practical. It feels like we're quitting, like we're saying to the one who has hurt us, "You win."

But let's think this through. Imagine someone has done you wrong. They did something to you that was unfair, something you didn't deserve, something that hurt you. Maybe a burglar vandalized your home and stole your computer or a neighbor didn't like how you parked, so they keyed your car or someone hacked into your phone and stole your identity. What are your options?

Are you familiar with Alexandre Dumas' famous 1844 novel *The Count of Monte Cristo*, detailing the egregious injustices suffered by the main character, Edmund Dantes, and the creative and extreme lengths Dantes went to in order to exact revenge? That classic and powerful novel illustrates one option, the option that comes so naturally to us: *you can take vengeance on them*. You can get them back. But most of us eventually come to understand that vengeance isn't a viable option. Life isn't a hockey game where, if someone checks you into the boards, you can check them back. If someone cuts you off when you're on the road, while part of you wants to do the same to them, you realize that you're likely only going to make a bigger mess of things; you're going to put yourself, your passengers, and other people in danger.

Here's what Lewis Smedes writes about the vengeance option: "The reason we cannot get even is that the victim and the victimizer never weigh pain on the same scale. One of us is always behind in the exchange of pain. If we have to get even, we are doomed to exchange wound for wound, blood for blood, pain for pain forever."[1]

In reality, most of our so-called "getting even" happens only in our private fantasies. We imagine what it might be like to get even, but we know we could never carry out our vengeful thoughts. And here's the kicker, as Smedes points out: our opponent feels no pain when we take revenge against him in our dreams; meanwhile, our fantasies become a catheter dripping a spiritual poison into our own system, making us more and more miserable as time ticks on.

Option number two when someone wrongs us is *bitterness*. We relive the hurt, picking at it like a scab until it bleeds all over again. We don't plot our revenge, because we know that would be wrong and impractical, so we simply sit and stew over the pain we feel. This is the option the majority of us choose. It is most certainly what I have chosen at various times in my life. I will be lying in bed, unable to sleep for one reason or another, when seemingly "out of the blue" comes the memory of the hurt someone has caused me, the wrong done to me. I become agitated, angry, frustrated. I relive the injustice of it all, the embarrassment in the aftermath. It's like a painful tooth that I keep biting down on just to see if it still hurts . . . which it does. But the old saying is true—*bitterness is a poison we drink while we wait for the other person to die.*

A group of people who became friends at the local gym often went out for coffee after their early-morning workouts. One of the more gregarious and congenial members of the group broke the news to the others that he was getting a divorce—his wife had left him for someone else. The group gave him their wholehearted support; they suffered with him and encouraged him. But the aggrieved husband refused to let go of his hurt. It was all he wanted to talk about, morning after morning after morning—how angry he was, how unfair it was, how cruel his ex-wife had been to him, how much he wished for her misery. He fed his bitterness day after day, until everyone in his group of friends drifted off, unable to stand being with him. Bitterness is not attractive; it has a way of driving away the people we need the most.

But there's a third option, what Jesus tells us is the option that is best not only for the one who did us wrong but for us who suffer unjustly—*forgiveness*. We can choose, by the power of God, to forgive the person for the wrong they have done to us. Ultimately, one of the most useful and most healing gifts we can give to ourselves is the gift of forgiveness. God not only commands us to forgive because it is right; He commands us to forgive because it is healthy. It is for our own good.

When I choose not to forgive, when I hold on to my anger and my bitterness and my resentment, I give the person who hurt me once the power to keep hurting me. It's as though I give them a bat and say, "Go ahead—hit me again." But when I forgive them, I put an end to the pain; I let go of the hurt. I unplug that catheter dripping the poison of bitterness into my soul. The best and healthiest way to live with the pain of an unjust hurt is not to plot revenge and it's not to nurse a grudge . . . it's to forgive.

Be Conscious of God

But *how* do I do that? How can I bring myself to forgive the drunk driver who crashed into my car or the vandal who broke into my house? Here's the real question: do I trust God to see that justice is done? Notice what Jesus's good friend Peter tells us about the way

Jesus handled the injustice He suffered: "When they hurled their insults at him, he did not retaliate; when he suffered, he made no threats. Instead, he entrusted himself to him who judges justly" (1 Peter 2:23). For me to reach the place where I am willing and able to forgive, I have to trust God—to trust that He is in control of all my circumstances, even the unfair ones, and to trust that He will ultimately do justice for all involved.

Okay, that's a big step. It's relatively easy to say, "Just trust God and forgive the perpetrator." But, in the words of the late Neil Armstrong when he first set foot on the moon, that's "a giant leap."

So let's start with a smaller step, before I take the giant leap of trusting God in my pain. I can simply *be conscious of God.* In fact, that's just what the Bible tells us to do: "For it is commendable if someone bears up under the pain of unjust suffering because they are conscious of God" (1 Peter 2:19). When you're suffering, you are mostly conscious of your pain. It's always there, nagging at you, taunting you, eating at you. But pain is not your only companion . . . so is God. Look for Him. Notice Him. Look for His fingerprints on your circumstances.

I love stories. I learn much better from them than from lectures. So I'm going to stop "lecturing" and tell you some stories. The first is a familiar Bible story of a young man who learned how to handle his unjust hurts in healthy ways when he became conscious that God was present in his life even when God seemed to be wholly silent. Then I'll tell you some stories from recent years to remind us that these truths God first taught us in the Bible can actually work for you and me.

The first story is told in the Bible's first book, the book of Genesis, and it's one of the most egregious examples of unjust suffering in recorded history. The victim in the story, who in turn becomes the hero, is named Joseph. It's a bit of a long story, which I will try to tell concisely, but it's well worth our time. Often when reading the stories of the Bible, we tend to skim over the details, but as Tim Keller points out in his book *"Walking with God through Pain and Suffering,"* the details of this story are particularly important.[2] And what the details of this story make very clear for us is that *God's fingerprints were on everything that happened to Joseph, even though much of what happened to Joseph was unjust and quite painful.*

"Time out," you say. "Are you suggesting that God sometimes composes the story of our lives in such a way as to cause us to suffer unjustly at the hands of hurtful people?" I understand why you would ask that, why that would bother you. But as counterintuitive as that sounds, as troubling as that sounds . . . yes. Since the Bible teaches us that God is sovereign—that God is in control of all the events of our lives—then we have to believe that He is sovereign over those events that cause us pain as much as we believe that He is sovereign over those events that bring us joy.[3]

So let's peek at the story, to see if this is really true.

Joseph was one of twelve sons, the favorite son of his father, Jacob, a fact that did not go over well with the others. In fact, Joseph's brothers detested him simply because their father loved him most. Joseph's father sent him off to check in on his brothers while they were away from home for their work. But instead of welcoming Joseph, his brothers grabbed him, stripped off his clothes, and threw him into a waterless well. Their initial plan was to kill Joseph, but they ended up selling him as a slave to a group of Midianites who "just happened" to be traveling by on their way to Egypt. When they got to Egypt, the Midianites decided to sell Joseph. And who should "just happen" to buy Joseph but Potiphar, the captain of Pharaoh's guard.

TAKE HOPE THAT GOD'S SILENCE
DOES NOT EQUAL GOD'S ABSENCE

By the way, there's one detail mentioned later in the story that you might be able to relate to. Later on in Genesis the brothers reminisce about their decision to sell Joseph into slavery, and they mention how Joseph—from the bottom of that well—begged and pleaded for his life . . . and they ignored him (Genesis 42:21). So let me ask you—*have you ever pleaded with God to intervene on your behalf and been met with silence?* Ever suffered unjustly and begged God to help you out . . . only to have your prayers bounce back like an e-mail with an invalid address? *It doesn't equate to God's absence.* Even though God doesn't come out and tell Joseph, "Don't worry, Joseph, I've got it all under control," the reality, as we will see, is that God did hear Joseph's cries and that God, in fact, had *everything* under control.

Things turned around just a bit for Joseph in Egypt. Joseph actually thrived as Potiphar's assistant; he bloomed where he was planted, as we say. But then more misfortune struck. Potiphar's wife tried to seduce Joseph, and when he ran from her, she decided to frame him. So even though Joseph did absolutely nothing wrong, he was thrown into prison and left to fend for himself. Except, we are reminded, he *wasn't* left to himself: "But while Joseph was there in the prison, the LORD was with him; he showed him kindness and granted him favor in the eyes of the prison warden" (Genesis 39:20–21). He was still in prison, mind you, but God had not abandoned him. In fact, God had Joseph right where He wanted him, even though his being in prison was a complete injustice. *God's silence does not equal God's absence.*

In his book *Soul Salsa*, Leonard Sweet describes the practice of a tribe of native Americans for training young braves.[4] On a boy's thirteenth birthday, he is taken to a dense forest to spend an entire night alone, left to fend for himself for the first time in his life. Every time a twig snaps, he imagines a wild animal ready to pounce. It is a long and anxious night. Hours go by before the first rays of sunlight break into the interior of the forest. Looking around, the boy who hasn't slept all night for fear of what might happen now sees flowers, trees, and the outline of a path. Then, to his great surprise, the boy spies the figure of a man standing a handful of feet away, armed with a bow and arrow. It is the boy's father, who has been there in the shadows, watching over his son, all night long.

God's silence does not equal God's absence.

At first blush God seemed to be absent from Joseph's story, and it may well feel that He is absent from yours. But the Bible makes it plain that God was very much present in all of Joseph's circumstances—as He is in ours—including those that seem wholly unfair. While in prison, Joseph became friends with Pharaoh's cupbearer and interpreted a dream for him. Later the cupbearer "just happened" to obtain his release from prison, and soon after that the cupbearer "just happened" to hear Pharaoh mention that he'd had some troubling dreams he didn't understand. The cupbearer told Pharaoh about Joseph, Pharaoh sent for Joseph, and Joseph explained the dreams. The dreams, Joseph explained, were from God.

That's another interesting fact showing how intimately God was involved in the details, the fact that God gave these dreams to Pharaoh. Pharaoh, obviously, didn't believe in Joseph's God. Pharaoh worshipped his own gods, like the sun god and the river god. Yet our God spoke, quite purposefully and miraculously, to this pagan ruler. God can do that, you know. *God can even use people who don't believe in Him to be helpful to us.* And God's message to Pharaoh was this: "The world is about to have seven years of prosperity, followed by seven years of crushing famine, so you'd better be prepared." Pharaoh, hearing Joseph interpret his dreams and explain all this to him, said, "Okay, Joseph, you're in charge. You handle this so we can survive the famine when it comes."

Don't Confuse a Pit Stop with the Pits

Now even before we finish this story, we discover another principle to help us live with our pain without becoming one—*don't confuse a pit stop with the pits.* Have you ever been in the pits—and been put there unfairly? Ever had a time when you were flat-out miserable, when everything was going wrong even though you had *done* nothing wrong? And you cried out to God and heard nothing in response, no matter how much you pleaded for God to intervene? We all know what that feels like; *it feels as if it's never going to end.* From where you sit, at the bottom of the pit, there appears to be no way out. The pit, for all you can tell, is permanent, which means your life is never going to get better, so everyone should just leave you alone and stop trying to cheer you up.

But a "pit stop" is temporary. We use the term "pit stop" to refer to those times when you pull off the road, fuel up, take a break, get something to drink, and then get back on the road. For a few years of my life, it felt to me like I was in the pits, like I was never going to get better—and there are still days when I feel that way. Joseph may well have felt the same when his brothers threw him in one pit and Potiphar threw him in another. He may well have felt that those pits were *permanent*. But they turned out to be *pit stops*—they were temporary. Joseph was miserable for a time, and his suffering was wholly unjust, but what he saw as a permanent pit, God intended as a temporary pit stop, as a means of preparing Joseph for something bigger and better.

Again, back to the story. (By the way, I know this is a long story—thirteen chapters. But *The Count of Monte Cristo* is 117 chapters and over 1200 pages . . . which is why most of us watch the movie instead of reading the book.) We're now into the famine, a famine that reaches the Promised Land far to the north of Egypt, where Joseph's family still lived. They heard there was food in Egypt, so they made the trip to see whether they could buy food. The brothers met Joseph, but they didn't recognize him. Eventually Joseph revealed his identity to his brothers, and you can imagine their reaction—*they were afraid.* Their fear was that Joseph would use his power to get his revenge on them for the years of pain and misery they unjustly caused him. And if this were a Hollywood movie starring Liam Neeson as Joseph, that's exactly what we'd expect to see.

But as he looked back on all the events of his life that brought him to where he then stood, Joseph recognized God's role even in the injustice he suffered—he was *conscious of God.* So instead of punishing his brothers, Joseph gave them the food they came for. He told them to bring the entire clan down from Israel for the duration of the famine. Joseph recognized that God put him in a position of authority in order to save thousands of innocent people. And so Joseph told his brothers: "You intended to harm me, but God intended it for good to accomplish what is now being done, the saving of many lives. So then, don't be afraid. I will provide for you and your children" (Genesis 50:20–21).

Joseph had a choice at that moment. He could have said, "God intended this for good so I could save many lives. And I'm going to save many lives . . . *but not yours.* " And if you're like me and kind of like the movies where the bad guy gets what's coming to him, maybe you're hoping Joseph did just that. But he didn't. He took the high road. He forgave. Why? Well, it wasn't because God sat him down and explained it all to him. *There's no indication at any point in this story that God ever explicitly revealed to Joseph His master plan behind Joseph's hardship and suffering.* But it seems what happened is that as Joseph took the time to reflect on all those "coincidences" in his life, he saw God's fingerprints over them all, and he chose to trust that God really did know what He was doing. *He chose to believe that even in His silence, God was very much present.* Joseph was "conscious of God."

So think about it. You've had bad things happen to you. In fact, evil has been done to you, evil you didn't deserve. You've been hurt, you've been betrayed, you've been lied about, you've been injured, you have suffered, *and it wasn't your fault.* And when you prayed, God was silent. And yet, might it be that God was with you all along, even when the pit stop felt like the pits? Don't forget Genesis 39:20–21: "But while Joseph was there in the prison, the Lord was with him." And might it be, if you stepped back a bit, if you looked carefully, that you could detect the fingerprints of God in some most unlikely places, orchestrating the seemingly random and often painful events of your life so as to do something wonderful and good both in you and through you.

TRUST THAT GOD IS
CONNECTING THE DOTS WE CAN'T

Now, let's be candid about this. The Bible doesn't promise that God is going to let us know on every occasion how He intends to use for good what others intend for evil. Clearly he gave Joseph enough information and insight so Joseph could connect the dots. *But it's very possible that in this lifetime, there will be many dots that seem to be nothing more than dots.* So here's our choice—will we still trust God to be God and to do justice? Will we take by faith God's promise to make everything work together for our good, even unfair things, even painful things, even miserable things that last a very long time? Because if we don't, our misery is sure to spill over onto everyone who gets close to us.

Douglas Groothuis is a brilliant Christian apologist and seminary professor who married an equally brilliant woman named Becky. But for much of their marriage, Becky has suffered terribly, first from fibromyalgia and then from primary progressive aphasia, a rare and cruel form of dementia that attacks the front of the brain before moving to the back. This disease is, as Groothuis describes it, "incurable, fatal, and horrible." Through it all—more than 25 years' worth of misery—Douglas and Becky have faithfully trusted their God. But they have struggled in vain to connect the dots. As Groothuis puts it, "Yet when I try to find the meaning in my wife's suffering, I come up dry and gasping. . . . I know there is a larger meaning behind it all, but I cannot parse it out day by darkening day."[5] God has not connected the dots for Douglas and Becky. And yet . . . they continue to trust God, to love each other, and to suffer virtuously.

I do not presume to suggest that it is at all easy to continue to trust God when our suffering is undeserved and it seems so very senseless or that it's easy to forgive our debtors as God has forgiven us. And yet, it is our best option and hope. Even when we can't connect the dots—which, quite honestly, is *most* of the time—we can trust the God who will.

When you boil down what the Bible says to all of us who suffer unjustly in this life, here's the message—*trust God, and do good.* Trust God's heart, trust His goodness and compassion. Trust that even though you can't see the big picture, the sovereign God is connecting the dots for good. Trust God, who sees all, who is the source of everything fair and just, to do justice for you and in the lives of those who have harmed you. It's what Jesus taught us to do, and it's what Jesus showed us how to do: "But if you suffer for doing good and you endure it, this is commendable before God. To this you were called, because Christ suffered for you, leaving you an example, that you should follow in his steps. . . . When they hurled their insults at him, he did not retaliate; when he suffered, he made no threats. Instead, he entrusted himself to him who judges justly" (1 Peter 2:20–21, 23).

TRUST GOD AND DO GOOD

And in addition to trusting God and forgiving those who hurt us, *do good.* Paul says it this way in Romans: "Do not repay anyone evil for evil. Be careful to do what is right in the eyes of everyone. . . . Do not take revenge, my dear friends. . . . Do not be overcome by evil, but overcome evil with good" (Romans 12:17, 19, 21).

So does all this work in real life, or does it only work in the stories of the Bible? I promised you more true stories, stories from our time and world. Here they are.

In 2005, Jameel McGee wasn't harming a soul when a police officer pulled him over and arrested him for possession of illegal drugs. McGee vowed it was all made up, that he was totally innocent . . . but he was convicted just the same. After McGee served four years in prison, the Benton Harbor, Michigan, police officer who arrested McGee recanted—the charge, in fact, *was* wholly made up. McGee's first thought? "I lost everything. My only goal was to seek him when I got home and to hurt him."[6] McGee wanted vengeance, and we can understand—when someone causes us pain, we want to be a pain to them.

But Jameel McGee "found" God while in prison, and so did Andrew Collins, the police officer, during his own stint behind bars for falsifying police reports and planting drugs. It's not hard to see God's fingerprints on what happened next. Both McGee and Collins "just happened" to get jobs at Cafe Mosaic in Benton Harbor, and before long they were working side by side. The issue could not be ignored, so they got to the point. Collins said he had no explanation and could only say he was sorry. And McGee forgave him. Collins and McGee have since become close friends. They often share their story of forgiveness and redemption—it is better to forgive, they've discovered, than to hang onto the hurt.

Kelly Putty was sixteen when two men in masks pulled her from her car and drove off into the woods.[7] Every time Kelly spoke, to beg them to let her go, they punched her in the face. They pulled the car over, and then, for the next few hours, they took turns raping Kelly. When their masks came off and she saw their faces, she assumed they were going to have to kill her. But they didn't.

The two men put Kelly back in the car and began driving. Oddly, they stopped to pick up the wife of the driver of the car from her place of work, and the wife took over the wheel. Within a few minutes, the wife drove them past the place where the men had abducted Kelly; Kelly could see the police investigating the scene. Kelly thought that was her chance—she began to scream and to beg the woman to stop the car and let her out. Thankfully, the woman did just that. Kelly jumped out of the car and ran to the police to blurt out her terrible story. In time, the men were arrested, tried, convicted, and sentenced to life in prison.

Life, understandably, was not the same for Kelly after that; the emotional pain was smothering, though she did her best to bury the pain and forget the past. She met a boy, Shane, who just happened to be a Christian, and they began to date. As a result of some of the injuries from her attack, Kelly became sick. She was told she had cancer and that she would be infertile. She began chemotherapy. And Shane, along with his church, began to pray for Kelly's healing.

The healing came quickly. Within weeks, Kelly's doctor was unable to find any evidence of cancer or of any scarring caused by her assault. As evidence of the extent of her healing, Kelly was pregnant, at the age of 17.

Shane was a follower of Jesus, but Kelly was not yet persuaded. She was still struggling with what happened to her, still struggling to let it go. She did attend church with Shane, though, whom she had married. One Sunday, when she was eight months' pregnant, the pastor explained how Jesus died on the cross to forgive mankind's sins. He explained how Jesus sets us free from shame and guilt and fear. And Kelly decided it was time to say yes to Jesus. Shane went to the front of the church with Kelly, and together they prayed with the pastor. Kelly's life began to change.

With the support of her husband and her church, Kelly made the decision to turn over her pain and her past to God and to forgive the men who had assaulted her. She often meditated on Jesus's words from the cross: "Father, forgive them; for they know not what they do" (Luke 23:34 KJV). It wasn't long before her ability to forgive was put to the test. In a neighboring church she was visiting one Sunday, the pastor asked everyone to come to the front of the church and to put a hand on the shoulder of the person in front of them and pray for that person. And when Kelly reached out, she noticed that the woman she had her hand on was the mother of one of her attackers, who had been in court supporting him throughout the criminal trial. Kelly hesitated . . . and then went ahead and prayed for her and her attacker. In Kelly's words, "God did a work in that moment and showed me the power of forgiveness."[8]

Trust God, forgive, and do good—which is exactly what Kelly did. Kelly and Shane now have seven children, two of whom they adopted from Ethiopia. In 2009, the Puttys founded Ordinary Hero[9], a child-advocacy organization whose mission is to inspire and empower ordinary people to make an extraordinary difference in the life of a needy child. When Kelly shares her story, she makes it clear that "forgiveness doesn't excuse the crime,"[10] but it does free the victim from her pain and resentment. Trust God, forgive, and do good.

Here's one more remarkable example of forgiving and doing

good. The book *Not by the Sword* tells the story of Larry Trapp of Lincoln, Nebraska, a longtime member of the Ku Klux Klan.[11] For years Trapp had targeted the Weissers, a Jewish family who lived in Lincoln, for persecution. He sent them pamphlets mocking how Jewish people looked and denying that the Holocaust ever happened. He made phone calls to their home, threatening to harm them. He bombed the synagogue where Michal Weisser was a cantor, which is something similar to a worship leader in a Christian church. But throughout the months the persecution took place, this Jewish family chose to respond to the evil by doing good, by returning love for hate. Then Trapp's health went bad. Long a diabetic, he became confined to a wheelchair and began to go blind. And Larry Trapp, by the way, had no family—at least no family that wanted anything to do with him. So what did Michael Weisser and his wife do? They took Trapp into their home to care for him; they made him part of their family. Won over by their goodness and compassion, Trapp renounced his membership in the KKK, got rid of his Nazi flags, and devoted himself to apologizing to all the Jewish and African-American people he had terrorized over the years. It is what it means to overcome evil with good. And it is what we as the people of God are called to do in response to those who intend to do us harm. Trust God, forgive, and do good—that's how we live with our pain without becoming one.

Nobody Caused Our Pain

But what are we to think and how are we to live when nobody caused our pain—not us nor someone else? How do we manage our pain when the only person we can possibly hold responsible for our pain is in fact . . . God Himself?

"When nobody did it:
Navigating the acts of God."

CHAPTER SIX

Our son was about four years old at the time. My wife was hard at work in her office when Ryan came running into the room. He had something to tell her—something important. Pausing to catch his breath, Ryan began with an announcement: "Nobody did it, Mom. Nobody did it." And then, before running back out of the room, Ryan said as calmly as he could, "I need a towel."

Now I'm sure you can put two and two together as quickly as Brenda did that day. Obviously there was some major spillage somewhere in our home, a spill that required something more than a paper towel to clean it up. And even before Brenda went to check out what happened, she was pretty sure that despite our son's assurances, *someone surely did this.*

Often in life we cause our own pain, sometimes by our misdeeds, sometimes by accident. Often the only one to blame for our pain is ourselves, which means that along with battling pain, we also suffer from guilt and shame. Fortunately, guilt and shame need not have the last word. For we who follow Jesus, grace gets the last word, grace that forgives our sin and heals our hurt. And while it's often true that we make our own messes in life, it's also true that there's a certain degree of suffering that comes our way not only through no fault of our own, but because of the meanness of other people. Someone steals from us; someone goes out of their way to hurt us. And when that happens, we struggle not only to handle the pain those people have caused us but also to handle the bitterness we feel in our hearts toward our wrongdoers, which can only be managed successfully by learning to extend to others the grace God has extended to us.

But my four-year-old son was actually on to something when he pronounced with such authority that "nobody did it." There are times in life when the pain we suffer isn't our fault, and it isn't someone else's fault. There are times when you didn't do anything wrong and no one else did either, and yet you still got hurt. And you've probably discovered this yourself—that can be a very unsatisfying place to be. We very much prefer to be able to point the finger at someone. We prefer to be able to explain to ourselves and to others why this bad thing happened to us.

Jeanne was diagnosed with breast cancer in 2010; it was Stage 3. She treated it aggressively—with chemotherapy, radiation, and surgery. She handled all the misery, pain, and anxiety with optimism, faith, and dignity. And remarkably . . . she beat it.

Then in 2014 she began to have pain in other parts of her body. At first her doctors weren't concerned, but when the pain persisted, they ran more tests and discovered that her cancer was back. It was in her spine, her abdomen, her lungs. Back for more treatment she went. Over coffee, Jeanne—still positive, still smiling—acknowledged that she will not "beat" this cancer, though she plans on living for some time. I'll tell you more of her story later; she's taught me a great deal about living in pain without becoming one. But my point here is simply this: Jeanne's cancer is not her fault, and it's not someone else's fault.

I've always been curious to learn how different religions and worldviews deal with the problem of pain. For example, the Buddhist view is that suffering comes from our unfulfilled desires and those desires are the result of the illusion that we are individual selves. Buddha taught that the solution to suffering is the "extinguishing of desire." This view is referred to by anthropologists as the "self-transcendent view."[1]

Hinduism takes a different approach to suffering, what anthropologists refer to as the "moralistic view."[2] This view, the "karmic" view, says that all pain and suffering stem from the failure of people to live rightly, either in this life or in a past life. If you are suffering now, karma teaches, it is likely your just desserts from your former life. In other words, your suffering—no matter what the immediate cause—is your fault.

But Jesus made it very clear that there are times when bad things happen in life and it's not your fault and it's not someone else's fault either. Do you remember the account of the man born blind, recorded in John 9? Here's how the chapter opens: "As [Jesus] went along, he saw a man blind from birth. His disciples asked him, 'Rabbi, who sinned, this man or his parents, that he was born blind?'" (John 9:1–2). The disciples wanted to know where to point the finger: do they point it at the man himself, or do they point it at the parents? Surely somebody did this; somebody had to be responsible. I doubt the disciples had ever heard of the doctrine of karma, but it almost sounds like that's what they're thinking.

After all, how else could the man's blindness at birth possibly been caused by his sin unless his sin was committed in a previous life? But Jesus makes it very clear that the man's blindness is nobody's fault: "Neither this man nor his parents sinned, . . . but this happened so that the works of God might be displayed in him" (John 9:3).[3]

Please don't assume that every bad thing that happens to you or to anyone else is caused by your sin or their sin. That's what I mean when I say "Nobody did it." I mean that it's no one's fault, that no one is morally to blame for what happened. You didn't get cancer or debilitating arthritis because you sinned. The tornado didn't level your home because you sinned. Sometimes bad things happen, and it's not because we messed up.

In his book called *The Question that Never Goes Away: Why?* author Philip Yancey talks about all the questions raised by the 9.0 earthquake that struck Japan on March 11, 2011, an earthquake so powerful that it jolted Japan's largest island a full eight feet closer to North America. The earthquake was followed, we remember, by a tsunami, a wall of water that reached a speed of 500 mph before it crashed ashore, leveling everything in its wake and taking approximately 18,000 lives. And in talking to people about the tragedy, Yancey found some people theorizing that the reason it happened was because so few people in Japan are Christians—less than 1 percent, by most accounts. In other words, the theory is that the tragedy happened because those folks were "worse" sinners. And as Yancey suggests, Jesus would say, "Wrong. It's not their fault. Nobody did it."[4]

But I know what you're thinking; you've been thinking it for a while. *Every time I say, "Nobody did it," you're thinking, "But what about God? Didn't God do it?* The earthquake—isn't that God? The cancer, the hurricane, the genetic disease—didn't they all happen on God's watch?" So what's our response? How do we navigate what the insurance industry has long labeled "acts of God?" How do we live with our pain when the only one we can think to blame for our pain is the God we love and worship?

WHAT WE KNOW ...
AND WHAT WE DON'T KNOW

First, let's address *what we know . . . and what we don't.* Second, let's get as practical as we can and talk about *what we can do . . . and what we shouldn't do.* So first, what do we know, and what don't we know when it comes to this problem of natural evil, of bad things that take place in our world that "nobody did"—nobody except for God Himself.

Here's what the Bible tells us we *can* know. It's not everything we'd like to know, but it's something. Let's start with a point we explored in a previous chapter—it's called "the curse," which is when God pronounced a curse on mankind and all of creation because of the sin of Adam and Eve. Romans 8 says, "For the creation was subjected to frustration, not by its own choice, but by the will of the one who subjected it, in hope that the creation itself will be liberated from its bondage to decay and brought into the glorious freedom of the children of God. We know that the whole creation has been groaning as in the pains of childbirth right up to the present time" (Romans 8:20–22 NIV84). One reason there is natural evil in our world is because creation is broken. According to the Bible, mankind broke it when Adam and Eve sinned. Our world is frustrated and subject to decay and disaster because it's damaged; the world we live in is not the perfect world God first created. Someday God will redeem this world, the Bible says, but that day is not yet, and until that day bad things will continue to happen.

Here's something else we can know: *sometimes natural evil is the work of the evil one.* Think again about the book of Job. Job was, the Bible says, a righteous man, an innocent man. But if you know the story, you know that horrible things happened to him and to his family. Among the tragedies that happened was this—his seven sons and three daughters were all killed when a mighty wind swept in from the desert and collapsed the house where they were having a party. Nobody did it; nobody was morally to blame. It was an act of nature, a mighty wind. But the text makes clear who was behind the wind: Satan, the evil one. We'll talk much more about that in a later chapter, but that's a piece of the puzzle; it's part of the bigger story. Sometimes natural evil is the work of Satan to wage war on God and His people.

But let me quickly add a *"we don't know"* to what we know. We almost never know when Satan is behind those kinds of tragic events. The book of Job is very much the exception, because the author comes out and tells the reader that those winds are the work of Satan. But remember this: Job himself didn't even know that. And that's how it usually plays out in our lives. Far more often than not, we simply aren't given that kind of specific information.

So part of the answer is that natural evil happens because we live in a fallen and fragmented world. Part of the answer is that it happens because we get caught in the crosshairs of a spiritual war between God and Satan. *And part of the answer is that God is, in fact, very much in control of everything that happens, but His intentions and His purposes and His designs are beyond our under-standing.* What the Bible wants us to know is that God is, to use a theological word, sovereign. God is in charge; He is in control. Nothing happens that is outside of God's ultimate control. Look, for example, at Amos 3:6: "When disaster comes to a city, has not the LORD caused it?" If you read through Amos, you'll find what kind of disasters God is talking about—ruined crops, drought, insects, horses that die, plagues. And through the prophet Amos, God also makes it very clear *why* He is afflicting the people of Israel with one disaster after another. It's to cause them to repent of their sin and return to their faith. In other words, God is using something painful and hard—a disaster—to accomplish something more important than His people's comfort and prosperity, and that is their salvation.

Here's another verse, this one from Isaiah. Through the prophet, God reveals this to His people: "I am the LORD, and there is no other. I form the light and create darkness, I bring prosperity and create disaster; I, the LORD, do all these things" (Isaiah 45:6–7). Or let's go back to the book of Exodus, where God is having a conversation with Moses. Moses is complaining that he's a bad choice to be a spokesman for God to the pharaoh, and this is how God responds: "Who gave man his mouth? Who makes him deaf or mute? Who gives him sight or makes him blind? Is it not I, the LORD?" (Exodus 4:11 NIV84).

Which brings us back to a story we started with—the man born blind. The disciples ask Jesus, "Whose fault it this? Who sinned—the man or his parents?" Jesus says, "Nobody did it; it's not the man's fault and it's not the parents' fault." But He doesn't stop there. Here's what he says: "Neither this man nor his parents sinned, . . . but this happened so that the works of God might be displayed in him" (John 9:3). Here's the point: God had a purpose behind this man's blindness, a good purpose. All his life the man had been in the dark about that purpose, until now, until Jesus gives him the gift of sight. And here's the bigger point; here's what we know; here's what the Bible tells us from beginning to end: *God is in control of everything that happens in our world, and His purpose and plan is to use it all for good.* Even disasters. Even blindness. Even deafness. Even . . . well, even the hard thing that happened to you.

But let's admit *what we don't know.* We don't always know *how* God is going to accomplish the good from the bad. In fact, I daresay that, most of the time, that's something we will not know until we get to heaven. And while that sounds like a cop out, think of it like this: it's an analogy theologians have used for many years to address just this issue. Parents, wouldn't you agree that there were times when your five-year-old asked you a question, even a very good question, and the reason you couldn't answer it *wasn't* that you didn't know the answer, but because your five-year-old simply wasn't yet mature enough to understand the answer? That's happened to all of us. And wouldn't you also agree that the gap between the intellectual abilities of a five-year-old and an adult pales in comparison to the gap between our intellectual abilities and the abilities of an infinite, almighty, omniscient God? In other words, just because we can't understand in the here and now how God might use something very bad to accomplish something very good, it shouldn't keep us from believing that our loving, gracious, omnipotent God can and will do just that, exactly as He's promised us He would.

I have a four-year-old granddaughter, McKenzie, who is very

smart, very verbal, and very inquisitive (and who can be a bit sarcastic when she doesn't think I'm giving her the right answer to one of her frequent questions). On election night, she was coloring in a map of the United States while her parents were watching the results, and she heard the commentators talking about the Electoral College. So she asked, "What's the Electoral College?" Now it could be possible to explain the Electoral College to a four-year-old; neither her parents nor I could figure out quite how to do it. But give McKenzie a few more years and I'm hopeful she'll be able to explain it to me.

There are many questions we have about God's ways in our world. But the mere fact that we are not capable at this point in time of understanding God's explanation does not mean that He doesn't *have* an explanation. And while I join you in wishing God would tell us far more than He does, I am grateful to worship a God who is far bigger than my abilities and understanding.

WHAT WE CAN DO . . .
AND WHAT WE SHOULDN'T DO

We've talked about what we know and what we don't know. But let's shift gears and focus on what we can do when natural evil strikes . . . and what we shouldn't do.

How do we live with the pain of natural evil; how do we handle it when there's no one we can blame for causing our pain other than our sovereign God? *Here's what we can do: complain.* If you're like me, that should come naturally. No one has to tell you to do that, do they? But specifically, what I'm suggesting is that if you want to live with your pain without becoming one, *take your complaints to God* and not to the people who are trying to love you and help you through your pain. Oh, I'm not saying that you shouldn't tell your friends your problems. I'm just saying that your complaints should be directed to the One who is in charge.

As you read through the Bible, you will find that the great men and women of the Bible did exactly that—they complained with great passion to God. Job did that. Read through Job and you'll read chapter after chapter of complaints. And after listening to Job for quite a long time, do you recall how God responded? Did God punish Job for his complaints? Did he strike Job dead? No. Job 38:1 says this: "Then the LORD answered Job out of the storm" (NIV84). It turns out that word "answered" is a significant word. In Hebrew idiom, to "speak to" someone indicates a one-way communication of an authority to an inferior, but to "answer" someone is to express a desire to enter into a dialogue.[5] And that's what God does in response to Job's complaints. Rather than lecturing Job, he invites Job into a dialogue. He welcomes Job's complaints. And commentators point out something else I never appreciated: God even gives Job the final word, in Job 42:1–6.

God invites us as His people to take our complaints directly to Him. He will not be offended. He will not strike us down. He will not lecture us. He invites us to come into His presence and enter into a dialogue with Him. So complain to your heart's content to the God who loves you. Talk to God from your gut. If you're not quite sure what to say, there are plenty of psalms you can use as examples (Psalm 10:1: "Why, LORD, do you stand far off? Why do you hide yourself in times of trouble?" Psalm 13:1: "How long, LORD? Will you forget me forever?" Significantly, nearly half of the Psalms are songs of lament.).

In the previous chapter, I referred to the story seminary

professor Douglas Groothius shared about the chronic illnesses suffered by his dear wife, Becky, and their struggle to find meaning in the midst of their misery. Douglas writes that one of the primary tools he's used to help him through their years of suffering is to bring his complaints to God through the laments of the Bible—in particular, the words of the book of Ecclesiastes. He writes that in the laments of Ecclesiastes he "found a light to shine on the path of pain."[6] Certainly there's more we can do, but for starters, we can take our complaints to God.

And here's what we shouldn't do: withdraw. That's the natural reaction of many of us to pain—we withdraw from everyone and everything. We pull away from the people who care about us. We try to go it alone. We stop going to small group meetings. We stop coming to church. We disengage from the things we used to do with our friends.

And it's the worst thing we can do.

One of the most important things we who suffer can do for each other is to communicate this truth to each other: *you are not alone.* In a study on pain, researchers recruited volunteers to test how long they could keep their feet in buckets of freezing water. They observed that when a companion was allowed in the room, the volunteer could endure the cold twice as long as those who suffered alone. Their conclusion was remarkable; just the presence of another caring person can double the amount of pain a person can endure.[7] As the Bible puts it, "If one part suffers, every part suffers with it" (1 Corinthians 12:26).

Katie Jo Ramsey is a young woman who suffers from ankylosing spondylitis, an arthritis that runs down the vertebrae of the spine, causing significant pain—pain that makes it an ordeal to get out of the house and go to church. But she makes herself go. Why? Because she knows "my body needs God and His body."[8] And she's exactly right—when our bodies are in pain, we not only need God; we very much need His body, the body the Bible calls the church.

In a letter to his protégé, Timothy, written from prison, Paul made an unusual request: "So do not be ashamed to testify about our Lord, or ashamed of me his prisoner. But join with me in suffering for the gospel, by the power of God, who has saved us and called us to a holy life" (2 Timothy 1:8–9 NIV84). You've probably asked your friends to do lots of different things with you: "Come to a movie with me." "Come to the game with me." "Go shopping with me." You've probably asked your friends to help you out from time to time: "Can you help me hook up my new washing machine?" "Can you help me move some furniture?" But have you ever asked anyone to do what Paul asked Timothy to do? Have you ever asked someone to join you in suffering? In the original language Paul used, that phrase "join with me in suffering" is the word *synkakopatheo*, which literally means "suffer together."[9] Paul is asking Timothy to partner with him in his pain. He doesn't want to go through his trial alone. He needs Timothy to join with him, to stand shoulder to shoulder with him.

But while we all know how helpful that can be, many of us are reluctant to reach out for help when we're in the middle of our suffering. The natural reaction of many of us toward suffering is to withdraw, to pull away, to go into hiding, to keep it all to ourselves. Maybe we don't want to bother anyone; maybe we think it's a sign of weakness; maybe we don't want people to see us cry; maybe we worry people will think our faith isn't very strong. I mean, if you're a strong Christian, you've got Jesus to help you—so why would you need anyone else's help?

And yet Paul, a giant of the Christian faith, needed help and wasn't ashamed to admit it. He needed his protégé to partner with him in his suffering. He needed to know that Timothy understood his pain, that Timothy was on his side.

I mentioned earlier my friend Jeanne, who has terminal cancer. Jeanne has an indomitable faith, an incredible husband and family, and gets a great deal of support from the Catholic Church where she's long been involved. But she also finds great strength in the support group she belongs to, a group of women she's met through her doctors who are on the same journey as she in dealing with a diagnosis of cancer. It helps, she says, to share their stories with each other; there's helpful information they share as well, about what works and what doesn't. In some respects, Jeanne says, being part of this group is another kind of pain, because as time passed, they have lost a number of their original members. But there is strength, comfort, and encouragement in being part of a group of friends who truly understand just what your struggle is all about.

I can't help but quote Joni Eareckson Tada on this point. Joni became a quadriplegic in the 1960s when she broke her neck in a diving accident. More recently, on top of her paralysis, she's had to battle cancer. She has had more pain in her life than I can imagine. I've pulled out some of her books during the last few years and reread some of the lessons she's learned about living with pain. This is something she wrote many years ago in her book called *A Step Further:*

We should never be alone when we suffer. I don't mean never for a minute or that we must not live in an apartment by ourselves. But we should never build a self-imposed wall around us that allows absolutely no one inside to see what we're going through and to hurt with our hurts.[10]

"We should never be alone when we suffer." Paul was in prison, chained and alone, so he wrote to his good friend Timothy and said, "Join with me in suffering." Most of the time, our friends can't take away our pain. They can't change our circumstances. But they can suffer with us and care for us and encourage us and comfort us. Don't shut them out. Your brothers and sisters in Christ care deeply for you and would be more than willing to partner with you in your pain if you would just ask.

When I was at my worst, my first instinct was to hide. Everything was hard, everything I did hurt, and I was completely embarrassed for people to see me look so pathetic. But I was blessed enough to have family and friends who wouldn't leave me alone and who were willing to just come over and feel bad with me. And I could see it in their eyes—they were genuinely suffering with me. Oh, my closest friends probably made fun of me when they left (for some reason it made me feel better to imagine them doing just that—it meant they believed I was was going to be okay), but at least while they were around me I could tell they were quite sincerely suffering right along with me. They couldn't fix me. They couldn't answer my questions. But they cared.

So let people care, because they really do. One pain I continue to battle is the nerve pain that makes my nights long and hard pretty much every night. So I got in the habit of getting out of bed and going downstairs so I could moan on the couch and not disturb my wife. But Brenda keeps telling me, I would rather listen to you in your pain and have you with me than have you go downstairs and moan to yourself. And while she can't make the pain go away, it really does help to have her hold my hand or pat me on the back and remind me that I'm not alone.

And neither are you. We are in this together. We are fellow strugglers. We don't have all the answers, but we do have each other, and we do have a great God who loves us and who promises to redeem our pain and hurt and suffering in ways far beyond our present ability to understand. Now, as Paul says, we see as through a mirror, dimly, but one day we will see face to face (1 Corinthians 13:12). And what we see when we see God's face will make all we've endured worthwhile.

DOES GOD WANT ME TO HURT?

While we're on this topic of natural disasters and the pain that can only come from God, maybe it's time to address another sticky subject—the pain the Bible says is by divine design. How can that be? I've always been told that God has a wonderful plan for my life. If that's the case, how could pain be part of God's plan? It sure doesn't strike me as wonderful.

"When pain is a calling: Embracing God's plan for my pain."

CHAPTER SEVEN

There's a branch of psychology referred to as vocational psychology, which is devoted to helping people find satisfaction and meaning in their work, and one suggestion some vocational psychologists have for people is "make your job your calling." What's a "calling"? In one sense, to have a calling to a particular job is to have a strong desire to do that job along with some sense that this is the job you are naturally gifted to do. But, for people of faith, calling is something a bit more; for people of faith to have a calling is to have a sense that God has in some way determined that this job or this path in life is what God in His wisdom and love has chosen specifically for you.

So what if I told you that pain and suffering is your calling as a follower of Jesus?

Yes, I imagine you've likely heard that before. And no, I'm not particularly thrilled with that thought either. At least not at first. But perhaps it makes sense to give God the benefit of the doubt, to trust that God would only call me to something that is ultimately for my own good.

A man named Saul discovered that to be true. Without a doubt the most dramatic conversion story in the Bible is that of Saul, described in the New Testament book of Acts. Saul was a brilliant person and one who had a strong distaste for those who followed Jesus. In fact, Saul made it his mission to put an end to Christianity, which he saw as a heretical movement contrary to the Judaism in which he was raised. And then one day, while traveling to Damascus to track down and arrest an enclave of Christians, Saul was struck by a bright light and a voice from heaven. The voice was that of Jesus, who said: "I am Jesus, whom you are persecuting. . . . Now get up and go into the city, and you will be told what you must do" (Acts 9:5–6). Saul was struck blind by the light and needed help to get to Damascus, where he went to wait for instructions.

At about the same time, Jesus appeared to one of His followers who lived in Damascus, a man named Ananias. The Lord explained to Ananias that his job was to go to Saul, pray for him to restore his sight, and give him further instructions. Ananias objected; he was well aware that Saul had come to Damascus to have him and his friends thrown in jail for their faith. So the Lord gave Ananias a glimpse into the bigger picture. Here's what Jesus said to Ananias about Saul: "This man is my chosen instrument to proclaim my name to the Gentiles and their kings and to the people of Israel." And then notice what Jesus says next: "I will show him how much he must suffer for my name" (Acts 9:15–16).

Saul later became known as Paul, the greatest missionary of all time. He took the message of the gospel from Israel to Turkey, Greece, and Italy. He wrote thirteen of the twenty-seven books of our New Testament. Most of his letters begin with the same introduction: "Paul, a servant of Christ Jesus, called to be an apostle . . ." (Romans 1:1). But the Lord made it clear to Paul right from the beginning that he was not only called to be an apostle, *he was called to suffer.*

So far we've seen that sometimes our suffering is our own fault and we have no one to blame but ourselves. Sometimes we suffer unjustly, when other people hurt us for no good reason. Sometimes nobody did it and we suffered anyway. *And sometimes we are called to pain.*

"So then, those who suffer according to God's will should commit themselves to their faithful Creator and continue to do good" (1 Peter 4:19). That, we've said, is how we want to live with pain, by trusting God and by continuing to do good. But notice what else this verse teaches us; it gives us another reason for *why* we sometimes suffer: "So then, those who suffer according to God's will . . . ." Sometimes our suffering is part of God's plan for our lives. It's not an accident; it's not a mistake. Some of our pain and our suffering is by divine design. God called Paul not only to be an apostle; God called Paul to suffer. And while we don't really want to hear it, Paul has news for us—*we are called to suffer too.*

Listen to what Paul writes in the book of Philippians, a letter Paul wrote while in prison for his faith: "For it has been granted to you on behalf of Christ not only to believe in him, but also to suffer for him, since you are going through the same struggle you saw I had, and now hear that I still have" (Philippians 1:29–30). Paul understood that it wasn't simply that suffering was his lot in life. He was called by God to suffer and calling was not unique to him. It is God's call and plan for each of us. In 1 Thessalonians 3:2–3, Paul writes this: "We sent Timothy . . . to strengthen and encourage you in your faith, so that no one would be unsettled by these trials. For you know quite well that we are destined for them." We are destined for trials, and the Bible is clear that God alone is in control of our destiny. Our trials are not accidents, and they are not mistakes; they are by divine design.

Now, my temptation is to show you verse after verse where the Bible tells us that pain can be a calling, that it is often God's will and plan that we suffer. But even if I convinced you of that, you'd still be left with the question of why. *Why* would God call us to suffer? Is God some kind of sadist? Does He want us to become masochists who learn to enjoy being in pain? Of course not. When someone you love hurts, don't you hurt? Sure you do. And that's how God is; He hurts when we hurt. In Isaiah 63 the prophet describes the suffering of God's people, and this is what he says about God's reaction: "In all their distress he too was distressed" (Isaiah 63:9). So if God hurts when we hurt, why would He ever call us to live in pain? And how does answering that question help us to live with pain without becoming one?

He Uses Our Suffering
to Shape Our Character

We learned in an earlier chapter that God changes our lives by changing our minds and that He can restore our souls in part by teaching us the truth about our pain. Here's more of the truth the Bible tells us about the purpose of our pain.

There are at least four reasons God has for bringing suffering into our lives . . . and you can probably guess the first one: *God uses our suffering to shape our character.*

If you have children or grandchildren, nieces or nephews, it might help to think of it this way. Is their character more important to you—or their comfort? Mind you, I'm not against any of my kids being comfortable; I don't pray for them to be cold, hungry, or miserable. But if it came down to a choice between their comfort and their character, I'd always choose their character. I care more about them being kind, gracious, courageous, and honest than I do about them being warm and full. Each of our three children went through some hardship and pain growing up, and as their father, I can honestly say that I suffered along with them. But I can also say that they wouldn't have developed the kind of character they have today without those hardships, and what matters to me in the long run is their character.

That's how God feels about us. Yes, He longs for us to be comfortable, healthy, and happy. But what He cares about far more is our character. And the hard truth is that there are certain qualities that can only be shaped by suffering of one kind or another.

In Romans, Paul writes, "Not only so, but we also glory in our sufferings, because we know that suffering produces perseverance; perseverance, character; and character, hope" (Romans 5:3–4). James, the brother of Jesus, writes this: "Consider it pure joy, my brothers and sisters, whenever you face trials of many kinds, because you know that the testing of your faith produces perseverance" (James 1:2–3). Now we understand that, but part of us wonders, "Isn't there some other way, some easier way, to shape our character than through suffering?" And when you think about it, you realize the answer is, no.

Think about growing in patience. Here's the definition of *patient*: "bearing or enduring pain, difficulty, provocation, or annoyance with calmness."[1] So let me ask you—how can you possibly grow in the ability to endure pain, difficulty, or annoyance if you never have pain, difficulty, or annoyance in your life? You can't! The fact is that there are certain character qualities we can't possibly develop without the experience of pain. As C. S. Lewis put it, "God allows us to experience the low points of life in order to teach us lessons that we could learn in no other way."[2]

And in fact, while Jesus lived a morally perfect life, did you know that even He needed suffering to help Him grow in His character? Listen to what the Bible says: "Son though he was, he learned obedience from what he suffered and, once made perfect, he became the source of eternal salvation for all who obey him" (Hebrews 5:8–9). Jesus learned obedience from what He suffered. And because Jesus wants us to grow to become just like Him, He gives us the chance to have the same experience of pain—growing pains.

Carol has been called to a life of pain. She has multiple sclerosis; she's had it for many years. It makes walking an adventure at times. She's had some spectacular falls. Being single and living alone only complicates the situation for her. Let's just say that this is not the life Carol would have chosen for herself.

I knew Carol before she was diagnosed with MS, before her divorce. She has always been fun; she's always made me laugh. But I have to say this, and Carol will be the first to admit it—Carol's suffering has made her a far sweeter, gentler person than when her health was better and her circumstances easier. In fact, the best evidence of this are the young kids in our church who love Carol as they love their favorite aunt. Carol's suffering has shaped her character.

Now here's an important point to keep in mind when we're talking about God using suffering to shape us: *It's not automatic.* Going through suffering doesn't automatically make you a better person. We've all known people—and maybe it was us (let's just say it—it was us)—who just got more impatient and grumpier and meaner, the more they suffered. As the saying goes, the same sun that melts butter hardens clay. If we want God to shape us in positive ways, we need to cooperate. We need to put ourselves in His hands and allow Him to bend us and mold us and shape us into the person He wants us to be.

I haven't always been particularly cooperative in that regard. Maybe it's part of why my pain has lasted as long as it has. But the person who knows me better than anyone on this earth, my wife, often tells me, "You're different now." (I think she means that in a good way.) And I am. My pain has made me a little less sarcastic and far more patient with people in pain. I feel with people much more deeply; I listen to people more easily. I am more grateful. Sometimes despite my resistance, God has used suffering to shape my character.

And when I choose to value God's shaping of my character over His catering to my comfort, when I learn to prize the strength of my soul over the ease of my situation, I will give less attention to my pain and more to the person I'm becoming. And here's what I've noticed about the people who do that—I like to be with them. Oh, I understand that they don't like their pain any more than I do. But it's not their focus; it's not the point of every story they share. Instead, what I hear from them is how they're growing— in their faith, in their empathy with the hurts of others, in their resolve to do good even though they feel bad. Yes, they ask me to pray for the healing of their hurts, but that's not all. Do you recall the prayer attributed to JFK? "Do not pray for easy lives. Pray to be stronger men." That's how they pray; that's how they ask me to pray. And though they are still clearly in great pain, they are not a pain to me. I am better for knowing them.

He Uses Our Suffering
to Share Himself

Here's a second reason God has for calling us to a life of suffering: *God uses our suffering to share Himself.* Have you noticed that one of the ways we get closer to each other is when we suffer through the same thing? That's part of the benefit of support groups, isn't it? You bond with this group of people who are going through what you're going through in a way you don't bond with people who are on the outside looking in. If you've suffered the loss of a child, you're likely to connect more closely with someone else who's lost a child than with someone who hasn't. Sports fans know this concept well. Some of you have suffered through decades of losing together and you are a tighter-knit group because of it. Men and women who have fought and suffered through war together know each other in a way nobody else knows them and are committed to each other in a way they're not committed to anyone else.

And one way we come to know God more intimately and personally is through suffering, because the Bible tells us that we and God share in suffering, that we suffer *together.* Paul wrote this: "I want to know Christ—yes, to know the power of his resurrection and participation in his sufferings, becoming like him in his death" (Philippians 3:10). That word "participation" is the Greek word *koinonia* which means "partnership."³ Paul understood that to really know Christ involved partnering with Him in His sufferings.

Here's how the Bible puts it: when we who follow Jesus suffer, we never suffer alone. Our Lord suffers with us. He doesn't just watch us suffer from a distance; He is in the trenches feeling our hurt and our pain right along with us. Do you remember Jesus's first words to Paul, then known as Saul? "Saul, Saul, why do you persecute me?" When Saul asked who was speaking, Jesus replied, "I am Jesus, whom you are persecuting" (Acts 9:4–5). Now Saul hadn't been physically persecuting Jesus, because Jesus had left the earth; Saul had been persecuting Christians. But according to Jesus, when he persecuted Christians, he was persecuting Jesus. Jesus was suffering *with* them; He was sharing in their suffering.

I was asked to pay a hospital visit to a man who had recently become paralyzed after suffering a fall at his home one night. He wasn't in much pain anymore, he explained, but he was struggling to adjust to his new reality. The days were better for him because, in addition to the nurses and therapists populating his ward, one or the other of his grown daughters was often able to keep him company. But it was the nights that were especially hard, he said, because that's when he felt the most helpless and, worse, the most alone.

Before I prayed with him, I read him a short passage I thought might offer a bit of comfort. Recognizing that he was a man of faith who knew the Bible better than I, I reminded him that Paul knew what it felt like to be alone. In the last letter Paul wrote before his execution, he explained, "At my first defense, no one came to my support, but everyone deserted me" (2 Timothy 4:16). And then Paul said this: "But the Lord stood at my side and gave me strength . . ." (2 Timothy 4:17). Notice what Paul does not say, I pointed out. Paul did not say, "It was *as if* the Lord was standing at my side." Paul's experience was that when everyone else deserted him, when he was all alone, Jesus showed up, stood by his side, and gave him strength. So that's what I asked Jesus to do for this faithful man that night—to show up and give him strength, to let him know that even if no staff or family member was around to help him, he was not alone. I can't tell you whether this man felt Jesus by his side every night after that, but there were some nights—in many ways still particularly hard nights—when Jesus "showed up," when His presence was certain even if not concrete, when His comfort was appreciable even if not tangible.

When you suffer, you too can know that you aren't suffering alone. The Lord is suffering *with* you and you with Him. And as you share in the Lord's suffering, you come to know the Lord more deeply and personally and intimately. In fact, you come to know Him in a way you couldn't unless you suffered. *So if you are serious about wanting to know God, here's the deal—suffering is part of the plan.* It is through our suffering that our God shares Himself with us, that He bonds with us in a personal way.

So how does that help me live with my pain? Would you agree that handling hardship is a little more manageable when you've got someone going through it with you? My wife and I tried to have our first child for nearly five years, but without success. We went to the doctor, we babysat for friends, we got a puppy, and we kept trying. Infertility can be hard on a marriage, especially if one partner feels like he or she is "responsible" or seems to feel the pain more deeply. In our case Brenda felt it more deeply than I did, and it added a layer of stress to our relationship.

Then one evening two of our closest friends, who had only been married a short while, stopped by to tell us their good news—they were pregnant. And being the mature Christian that I was, it made me mad. Oh, I wasn't mad in front of them. But once they left, after we celebrated with them as best we could, I got mad in front of my wife. And her response was to hug me tighter than she ever had and to tell me how much she loved me and appreciated me (who knew getting mad would make me the best husband in the world!). Finally she felt it—we were partners in our pain. And that experience of sharing our pain made our relationship all the stronger and all the sweeter. Eventually Brenda and I had three children, and we love them dearly. But the connection she and I made with each other in that very painful season of life . . . I wouldn't trade it for anything.

I imagine you would love to know God better, more personally; I believe we all do. It turns out that one of the most effective ways to connect with God is to participate with Him in pain. The best way to live with pain without being a pain is to have a partner in your pain. And there is no better partner than God.

HE USES OUR SUFFERING TO SHOW HIS GLORY AND GRACE

A third reason God purposely brings suffering into our lives is this: *He uses our suffering to show us His glory and grace.* This is one of the themes of the book of 2 Corinthians. Listen, first, to what Paul writes in chapter 4: "But we have this treasure in jars of clay to show that this all-surpassing power is from God and not from us. We are hard pressed on every side, but not crushed; perplexed, but not in despair; persecuted, but not abandoned; struck down, but not destroyed. We always carry around in our body the death of Jesus, so that the life of Jesus may also be revealed in our body" (2 Corinthians 4:7–10).

God's ultimate goal, the Bible tells us, is to save as many people as possible, to rescue all He can from the power and penalty of sin. Now He's given us the Bible to explain to us the good news of the gospel. You might have noticed, however, that most of our friends don't read the Bible. But they do "read" us. They watch how we live and how we talk and how we respond to hardship. So one way God reveals His glory and His power and His grace to the world around us is through our suffering. When people who know us see that we are hard pressed on every side but not crushed . . . when they see we are perplexed but not in despair . . . when they see we are struck down but not destroyed . . . they will see God's glory and power and grace at work in us.

Some of you have suffered through a divorce. I'm not sure I've ever seen a divorce that wasn't accompanied by the word "messy." Even the "cleanest" divorces are hard, and some of the ones I've witnessed have been torturous. And sometimes, when you're going through that, you sort of want to hide from people; you don't want people to know what you're going through. But the fact is that there are people all around you, both non-Christians and Christians, who are going through the same thing and who desperately need to see God's glory and power and grace in your life to give them hope that God can help them through their own pain. They need to see that you are hard pressed on every side but that because of the grace of God, you are not crushed. A pastor I know went through a particularly unpleasant divorce, made all the more disconcerting because of his vocation. To begin with, I would not say he handled it well, though I make no promise that I would handle it any better. But as time went on, he very much rose to the challenge. It was evident to many who knew him, both in the church and in our community, that God's grace was making a difference in his life. So let's learn to take a small measure of pride—as hard as that is—that our God has chosen to use us as His means of revealing Himself in all His glory and grace to the watching world. You'll still be living with pain, but instead of being a pain, you'll be a billboard for God's power to redeem our brokenness.

HE USES OUR SUFFERING
TO SHAKE EVIL'S GRIP

Here's a fourth reason God calls some to a life of suffering (and there are surely more reasons that God hasn't yet told us about): *God uses our suffering to shake evil's grip.* Now we're going to spend the next chapter exploring this in more detail, but let me at least briefly introduce the topic. One of the ways God uses to defeat Satan and evil is through suffering. And this is very much by design; it is part of God's plan. And the clearest and best example in the Bible is, of course, the life and death of Jesus Himself.

In Acts 2 we read Peter's sermon on the Day of Pentecost, his first recorded attempt to explain the gospel to his countrymen. Notice what he says about Jesus: "This man was handed over to you by God's deliberate plan and foreknowledge; and you, with the help of wicked men, put him to death by nailing him to the cross. But God raised him from the dead, freeing him from the agony of death . . ." (Acts 2:23–24). Did you catch whose plan it was that Jesus be condemned to an agonizing death? It was God's. God the

Father called Jesus to suffer horrible pain. Jesus's torture and death wasn't an accident or a ghastly mistake—it was part of the divine design for His life. And you don't need me to tell you what God's purpose was in calling His Son to a life of pain; it was to shake the grip of evil on mankind. It was to pay for our sins, to make salvation possible, and to defeat death. Here's how the Bible explains it in Hebrews: "Since the children have flesh and blood, [Jesus] too shared in their humanity so that by his death he might break the power of him who holds the power of death—that is, the devil—and free those who all their lives were held in slavery by their fear of death" (Hebrews 2:14–15). Jesus was called to suffer terribly, and it was through His suffering that Jesus was able to shake Satan's grip on humanity and set us free from the fear of death.

As I said, we will talk much more about this in the next chapter, about how God uses our suffering to shake evil's grip. But let's make sure we've got a grip on the big point of this chapter, which is this—*as followers of Jesus, we are all called to suffer.* It is part of what we signed up for when we said yes to Jesus. It's exactly what Jesus said. Remember this hard saying of Jesus? "Whoever wants to be my disciple must deny themselves and take up their cross daily and follow me" (Luke 9:23). In essence, Jesus says, *"Embrace hardship."* The Bible's coaching to us who suffer, which is all of us, is to embrace God's plan for our pain. Again, that doesn't mean to be masochistic about it. But let's accept the facts. First, God has called us to experience pain in this life, and second, God has a plan for our pain. *Your pain is not pointless.*

We've seen four ways the Bible says God uses our pain, and there are certainly more than that. Part of embracing our pain is to trust that God has a purpose and a plan for our pain, even if He doesn't choose to reveal that purpose to us. I wish that every experience of pain came with a letter from God explaining the point behind it, but sadly I've never gotten one of those letters, and I imagine you haven't either. But this is what we believe, because this is what the Bible teaches. Our pain is not pointless. God has a purpose for our pain. We can live with pain without being a pain when we embrace God's plan for our lives, a plan that includes pain.

Maria has done that. Maria is one of the smartest people I've ever met. She is fluent in a handful of languages, so much so that one of her vocations is to translate books written in English into a variety of European dialects. She is an astute theologian, widely read and quite experienced as a teacher. She is a missionary and a Bible study leader. And she has suffered as much as anyone I've ever known.

Maria was born with severe bone deformities. As a child growing up in Communist Romania (one of eleven children), she could not walk or ride a bike, so she dragged herself along the ground to get to school. She had scores of surgeries growing up; she's had pain in her back and her hips for as long as she can remember. She is very short. When she stayed at our home on a trip through California, she good-naturedly allowed us to measure her, and she's closer to four feet than five. Maria suffers from a rare disease known as osteogenesis imperfecta, which is painful, debilitating, and embarrassing.

Maria would much prefer not to be in pain; she would rather be taller and able to drive and run and jump. She would like to not have more surgeries in her future. But what I have learned from my time and communication with her is that Maria has embraced God's calling on her life, a calling that includes a significant amount of pain and suffering. She believes with all her heart that as long as she continues to trust and serve God, He will continue to work everything in her life for her good, even those things that are incredibly hard.

You probably know this verse: "And we know that in all things God works for the good of those who love him, who have been called according to his purpose" (Romans 8:28). Yes, God calls each of us to pain, but He always has a plan, and His plan is to work all things together for our good when we love Him and trust Him and live for His purposes.

Katherine Wolf was a beauty queen, a wife, and a mother of a six-month-old boy when, at the age of 26, she suffered a massive brain-stem stroke that nearly took her life.[4] The stroke left her unable to walk, talk, or swallow, along with double vision, right-ear deafness, and right-side facial paralysis. But while Katherine's life is undeniably tragic in many ways, there is also undeniable good that has come from her suffering. Five years after her stroke, Katherine and her husband gave birth to a new ministry called "Hope Heals" that serves those who struggle with physical disabilities, a ministry that has given hope to many thousands of fellow sufferers.[5] Among the truths Katherine shares through her ministry is this—that "hard" and "good" are not mutually exclusive to each other, that things can be very good and very hard at the same time. And this former beauty queen is also quick to point out something. Far more important than our outer beauty, which fades for all of us in time, is our inner beauty, our character, that follows us into eternity. Katherine lives with pain, but she is not one—she is a woman of beauty, faith, and grace.

Sometimes Pain Is Just Plain Evil

But there is a pain, the Bible says, that is just plain evil. Does God work that pain together for our good as well? What's the truth about pain that is just plain evil, and how do we manage it without becoming a pain? That's next.

"When pain is just plain evil: Engaging the enemy."

CHAPTER EIGHT

I know I'm a pastor and that I preach and teach about the supernatural every week, but I have to admit something to you—I am often a little slow when it comes to taking seriously the work of Satan and his demons. Part of it is a reaction to some people I knew growing up who had a tendency to blame everything they didn't like on Satan. If the weather was too hot or too cold, it was Satan's fault. If they didn't get a convenient parking spot, it was the work of Satan. If the wrong candidate won the election, it was clearly the hand of Satan. And my thought when I would listen to them was usually, "Really! Don't you think there might be an explanation for the cold you caught other than Satan's supernatural intervention?"

But over the years I've become more of a believer. No, I don't think Satan controls the outcome of every football game, and I don't think every problem with my car can be attributed to him messing with my life. But I have come to conclude that there are times in life *when the pain we suffer is just plain evil.*

The primary reason I believe that is because Jesus said so. In the book of Luke, we read about Jesus's encounter with a woman who had been crippled for eighteen years. Luke tells us "she was bent over and could not straighten up at all" (Luke 13:11). Jesus healed her, but he healed her on the Sabbath, which made certain people mad—people who insisted that there were six days for healing but the Sabbath was to be a day of rest. Listen to Jesus's response: "You hypocrites! Doesn't each of you on the Sabbath untie your ox or donkey from the stall and lead it out to give it water? Then should not this woman, a daughter of Abraham, whom Satan has kept bound for eighteen long years, be set free on the Sabbath day from what bound her?" (Luke 13:15–16). Did you notice where Jesus points the finger? He points it directly at Satan. He says Satan is the one who has kept this woman physically disabled and in significant pain for eighteen years. Her pain was just plain evil.

So here's what we want to know. First, is there any way to know whether *our* pain is just plain evil? Second, where is God while Satan is attacking His people; why would God ever allow Satan to cause us pain? And third, how do we manage the pain that is just plain evil; how do we live with that kind of pain without becoming a bigger pain to those who care about us?

SOME PAIN IS JUST PLAIN EVIL

Let's start by making sure that our beginning premise is accurate biblically: Is it really true that some pain is just plain evil, that some of our pain is in fact the work of Satan? And if it is, then we want an answer to the next question we're all wondering—where is God in this? What is God doing while Satan is tormenting and bedeviling God's people?

From beginning to end, the Bible makes it clear that we as the people of God are in a battle with Satan. We see the first glimpse of the conflict in the third chapter of the Bible, when Satan tempts Adam and Eve in the garden, and the struggle continues right through the very last book of the Bible, the book of Revelation, where the Apostle John reveals to us that Satan has declared war on you and me as followers of Jesus (Revelation 12:7–9, 17). I appreciate that there are many images in Revelation that are confusing to us, but in Revelation 12 John spells things out for his readers quite clearly, and this is his point—Satan, out of his anger toward God, is at war with all who follow Jesus. He intends to do us harm. He wants to hurt God by hurting us. And because we're in a war with Satan, we sometimes suffer pain and heartache. Sometimes pain is just plain evil.

You're probably familiar with this next example. In 2 Corinthians 12, Paul talks about his "thorn in the flesh," a thorn he pleaded with God on three occasions to remove from him. In the next chapter I'll talk more about God's response to Paul's prayers, but notice what Paul says about the source of the thorn: "In order to keep me from being conceited, I was given a thorn in my flesh, a messenger of Satan, to torment me" (2 Corinthians 12:7). Who was behind Paul's thorn? Satan. Satan brought a thorn of some kind into Paul's life not just to annoy him, but to torment him. Sometimes pain is just plain evil.

Of course the best example of this comes from what most Bible scholars believe is the oldest book in the Bible, the book of Job. Job is the most righteous man on earth, and he's very prosperous. Satan approaches God and says, in essence, "I bet you that if you take away Job's prosperity, he'll turn his back on you. I bet that if life gets too hard or too painful for Job, he'll give up his faith." And God says, "I'll take that bet. Do your worst, but you can't take his life." So Satan goes to work. He sends a bunch of bandits who steal Job's oxen and donkeys, which are the source of his livelihood. Then Satan sends a fire that kills Job's sheep. Then he sends another group of thieves who make off with Job's camels. Then Satan sends a strong wind that blows a house down and kills Job's seven sons and his three daughters. Then we read this: "So Satan went out from the presence of the LORD and afflicted Job with painful sores from the soles of his feet to the crown of his head" (Job 2:7). Satan afflicted Job and caused Job to suffer pain from the bottom of his feet to the top of his head. That pretty much covers it, I would say. Sometimes pain is just plain evil.

How Can We Know?

But what about *our* pain? How can we know if our pain is just plain evil?

Here's my less-than-satisfying answer: I don't know. I don't find anything in the Bible that helps us to definitively discern whether Satan is responsible for our pain. With that said, I believe there are times when we can logically conclude from the totality of circumstances that our suffering is just plain evil. Randy Alcorn more than hints at this in his book *If God Is Good,* in raising such truly awful events as the death camps of Nazi Germany and the Cambodian killing fields. Alcorn then writes more personally, "Three times in my life, each unexpected, I have faced the palpable presence of supernatural evil. In each case it was distinctly not of this world."[1]

Here's an analogy that might help from my days as a lawyer. The issue before the Supreme Court in the 1964 case of *Jacobellis v. Ohio* was whether a particular movie was "obscene" under state law. In ruling that the movie was not legally obscene, Justice Potter

Stewart famously wrote that he might never be able to intelligibly define what constitutes hard-core pornography. But, he concluded, "I know it when I see it."

Can we "know it when we see it" when it comes to discerning whether our pain is just plain evil? That's probably not the most reliable test to use. And yet it does seem that God is able to give us some sense of what is from Him and what is from Satan. He does command us to "test the spirits to see whether they are from God" (1 John 4:1), so perhaps it makes sense that God would enable us to "test" whether Satan is the source of our pain.

More often, I believe, we simply won't know for a fact that Satan is the cause of our pain unless God in His grace chooses to reveal it to us. But the larger point remains: God wants us to know how to think about our pain, and one thing He has chosen to make very clear is that there are times when pain is just plain evil.

Sometimes God Allows what He Hates to Achieve what He Loves

But where is God while all this is going on? Why in the world, if God is sovereign, does God allow Satan to cause the people He loves so much pain and misery?

And notice how I said that—God "allows" Satan to cause us pain. Satan is not free to run amok in our world. Satan doesn't have the power or authority to do to us whatever he wants. The Bible makes it clear that Satan must get *permission* from God to do what he does, just as Satan got permission from God to do what he did to Job. Do you remember a conversation Jesus had with Peter shortly before His arrest? Jesus said to Peter, "Simon, Simon, Satan has asked to sift all of you as wheat" (Luke 22:31). Satan's bad acts in our world, acts which are just plain evil, are done only with God's permission.

And that doesn't really sound very good, does it? That makes God sound as if He's less than the compassionate, gracious God we tell people He is. But think about it this way. What if Satan acted solely on his own? What if Satan wasn't in any way limited by God? Here's how one author puts it: "If God didn't control evil, the result would be evil uncontrolled."[2] As bad as things can be sometimes, they could be far worse if God was not at the wheel, so to speak.

Did you ever play dodgeball as a kid? Most of the time I played it in gym class when a teacher was watching or at recess when the yard-duty person was in charge. But once in a while we would get to play when no adult was around to supervise. And what I remember is that those unsupervised games were far more vicious than the supervised games. The rule, of course, is that if you hit someone with the ball once, they're out. Another rule is that you can't purposely hit a person in the head. But did we follow those rules when the teacher was out of the picture? Not usually. We wouldn't hit the person just once—we'd hit him with every ball in the gym. And I can assure you that the guys throwing the balls at me were using my head for a target.

If God was not sovereign, if God was not in total control of our world, our pain and suffering would be far worse than it is. *"If God didn't control evil, the result would be evil uncontrolled."*

But there's still that nagging question of why God allows it at all. Why does God ever say yes to Satan? What possible reason could a loving, gracious God have for giving a wholly evil being the right to cause us pain and misery? Suppose someone came to me and asked, "Can I push your one-year-old granddaughter down so she gets a bloody nose and a knot on her head?" Would you think I was a good grandparent if I said, "Sure, go ahead, but don't break any bones." I have a hunch that would be the last time I ever got to babysit my grandchild. You would think me a bad grandparent for allowing my granddaughter to suffer pain, even if the pain was limited. So how is it that our God, who we believe loves us with all His heart, would ever grant Satan permission to cause us pain?

Let me give you the principle that theologians offer us, and let's see if this makes sense. Here's the principle: *sometimes God allows what He hates to achieve what He loves.* Here's an example that Dr. James Dobson writes about in his book *When God Doesn't Make Sense* that I think illustrates the point. Dobson's son Ryan was only three years old and had a terrible ear infection that just wouldn't get better. The specialist told Dobson that the only way to treat the situation was to pull off a scab that had formed on his son's eardrum. He warned Dobson that this was very painful but very necessary. So Dobson did what he had to do–he sent in his wife to hold Ryan down while the doctor pulled off the scab. But his wife wasn't strong enough to hold their son, so she went out and sent Jim in. Jim did his best, but little Ryan squirmed out of his arms, which prompted the doctor to give Jim a tongue-lashing and to tell him to man up. So Jim summoned all his strength to wrap his large frame around his small son while the doctor performed this painful procedure on his three-year-old. And the whole procedure took place in front of a large mirror. Jim and his son could see the other's face, and Jim says the worst part of the whole event was seeing the sense of betrayal in his son's eyes and being unable to explain to him that it was for his own good.[3]

Sometimes God allows what He hates to achieve what He loves.

Sometimes God allows Satan to bring us pain, even great pain, to achieve what is ultimately for our good and for His glory. Why doesn't God explain it to us? That would help, wouldn't it? It would still hurt, but at least it would make it easier to keep the faith. But like we've said before, just as it is sometimes impossible for a parent to explain what he's allowing to happen to his three-year-old son, sometimes it's impossible for our omniscient God to explain His ways to creatures as limited as we are.

Of course, the best example of this principle is the most obvious—the crucifixion of Jesus. We looked at this verse in the last chapter, where on the Day of Pentecost, Peter said this to the crowds in Jerusalem: "This man [Jesus] was handed over to you by God's deliberate plan and foreknowledge; and you, with the help of wicked men, put him to death by nailing him to the cross" (Acts 2:23). There's no doubt that God hated seeing His Son nailed to a cross and put to death. But He allowed it to achieve what He loved—your salvation and mine. *Sometimes God allows what He hates to achieve what He loves.*

THE SUPERNATURAL WORLD IS WATCHING HOW WE HANDLE OUR PAIN

So here's our next question—what possible reason does God have for allowing Satan to inflict pain on us? What is the good He hopes to achieve by allowing us to suffer what He hates?

We can imagine a number of good things that might be behind God's mysterious ways, but let me focus on just one that you might not have thought about before. This is a truth I first learned over thirty-five years ago at a conference with Edith Schaeffer, the wife of author Francis Schaeffer, which she wrote about in her book simply titled *Affliction*.[4] Her explanation came up in the context of a question that went something like this: "What about the pain we suffer that nobody sees? I can see how it might honor God if people saw us keep the faith while we endured suffering publicly, but what possible value is there for me to bear up under pain when no one is watching?" And Edith Schaeffer's response was, *"There is always someone watching."*

Think again of the story of Job. Who was the primary audience to Job's suffering? Yes, he had some less-than-helpful friends who told him, quite wrongly, that his suffering must have been caused by his sin. But they weren't the primary audience. The primary audience was a supernatural audience; it was Satan and his demons and God and his angels. Remember the "bet"? Satan bet God that Job would renounce his faith if Job lost all the good things God had given him. But God had faith in Job; He believed Job would stay true. And while Job struggled, in the end Job proved God right. Who did Job prove God right to? To the supernatural world— to the heavenly realm.

And Edith Schaeffer's theory is this: just like God bet on Job, God is betting on us. God is demonstrating to the watching supernatural world that no matter what Satan throws at us, we will hang tough and trust God.[5] There's a verse in Ephesians that's kind of a mouthful but supports this theory that the supernatural world is watching us: "[God's] intent was that now, through the church, the manifold wisdom of God should be made known to the rulers and authorities in the heavenly realms" (Ephesians 3:10).

Since September 10, 2012, when I had my last hip surgery, I wake up numerous times every night in pain. One of the frustrating parts of the pain is that it makes no sense to me or to my doctors.

I have no explanation for it. It's like an electrical shock that spreads through most of my body. Some nights it's not as bad as others, and some nights—many nights—it's just miserable. I often have bad dreams along with the pain, as my subconscious tries to make sense of it, so I'll dream that I'm being eaten or beaten or operated on. Brenda points out that I talk to myself a lot at night, and she's right. And if she happens to be awake when I do that, she hears me say something like this: "God, this makes no sense . . . God, what's the point of this?"

Well, maybe this is the answer, or at least part of it.[6] Maybe the point is to demonstrate to the watching supernatural world that even if you short-circuit the body of one of God's kids every single night and make him wish he didn't ever have to sleep again, he would still trust God. There may certainly be other reasons of God's, to allow what He hates to achieve what He loves, but it's possible that in my case, this is the reason.

By the way, Jesus taught us Himself that the supernatural is very much interested in what goes on in our lives here on earth. Do you remember in Luke 15 when Jesus said this: "I tell you, there is rejoicing in the presence of the angels of God over one sinner who repents" (Luke 15:10)?

The contemporary singer Lady Gaga wrote a hit song in 2013 called "Applause." The primary lyric simply says, "I live for the applause."[7] Think about it like this: would it make the experience of pain more meaningful to you if, at the end of the day, thousands of people stood and applauded you for hanging tough in your hard times? I kind of think it would. Or imagine this—you're playing for the 49ers (or any opposing NFL team) at Seattle, where the fan noise gets up to 135 decibels. What would be the sweetest sound in the world to you as an opposing player? It would be the silence of the crowd, because that would mean you just did something to beat their team. That's much like what's happening when we stand tough in our hard times—we're silencing the watching enemy and eliciting the cheers of the onlooking angels.

How Can We Handle the Enemy?

Here's the last question: how do we handle this enemy? And how do we help each other in handling this enemy? How do we live with our pain without becoming one when the pain is just plain evil?

First, let's look quickly at how we can help our fellow sufferers. Paul offers this: "I urge you, brothers and sisters, by our Lord Jesus Christ and by the love of the Spirit, to join me in my struggle by praying to God for me" (Romans 15:30). A friend pointed out to me that the Greek word Paul uses here is *sunagonizomai*, which literally means "to struggle with me"[8] (we get our English word "agonize" from *agonizomai*). Paul is asking his friends to join him in his struggle by agonizing with him how? *In prayer.* When people share their stories of pain with us, we can help them by agonizing along with them in prayer. After all, if their pain is part of a spiritual war, as Revelation says it sometimes is, then it makes sense that we use spiritual methods to do battle. So when you tell your friend in pain, "I'll pray for you," it's not a way of telling them to quit their whining because you don't want to hear it anymore. You're telling them, "I'm in this with you. I'm joining the battle. I will *struggle with you* against the enemy. I will *agonize with you* through this trial. I am going to war right alongside you." We should never say, "Well, all I can do is pray for that person," as if that's nothing.

It's everything. Let's agree, we fellow sufferers, that we will join in others' struggles by praying for each other. Let's pray for grace, for hope, for deliverance, for healing, and for victory.

I had just come back to work after my last hip-replacement surgery. I was still in pain, feeling very sick and weak and, frankly, fairly hopeless. A good friend of mine from our church came over to take me to lunch and to see how I was doing. We walked to a restaurant close to my office, got our food, and had started to eat and catch up with each other, when out of the blue, my pain and sense of hopelessness got the better of me. I started to cry. I'm not sure what I would have done had I been on the other side of the table, watching my friend and pastor break down in public like that. But Chris didn't hesitate. He walked over to me, put his hands on my shoulders, and prayed for me. He didn't care that people were looking at us, wondering what might be going on. For about three minutes, Chris agonized with me in prayer, entreating our good and gracious God to intervene and give me comfort, strength, and hope. And while the pain didn't go away, I can assure you that Chris's prayer helped redeem my day and restore my soul.

Are you struggling to manage your pain, the pain that may be just plain evil? Find a prayer partner, a person of faith who will agonize with you by praying for you. It can make all the difference in the world.

Last, look at what Peter says at the end of his first letter about engaging the enemy when our pain is just plain evil: "Your enemy the devil prowls around like a roaring lion looking for someone to devour. Resist him, standing firm in the faith, because you know that the family of believers throughout the world is undergoing the same kind of sufferings" (1 Peter 5:8–9). Resist the enemy, Peter says, when your pain is just plain evil. Don't give in.

It was on one of those nature shows on TV. The place was Africa, and we were learning how a lion catches its dinner. When a lion comes across a herd of prey, he doesn't go charging into the herd—the herd could quickly defend itself by turning on him en masse. So the lion circles the herd, looking for the lame, the weak, the injured. And when he's chosen his mark, the lion goes to work, skillfully separating his target from the herd, isolating the wounded and weak. Then . . . he pounces. Which is often how Satan, who prowls around like a roaring lion, attacks us. He waits for us to withdraw from those who love and support us; he separates us from our friends and fellow sufferers. Then . . . he pounces.

Part of what gives you the courage to resist the devil is knowing that you aren't alone; you belong to a family of believers all around the world that suffers as you do. Don't withdraw. Stay connected; stay engaged with your family of believers; let them surround you and protect you with their presence and their prayers.

But that's not how Peter ends this section; recall what he says next. We've seen this verse before: "And the God of all grace, who called you to his eternal glory in Christ, after you have suffered a little while, will himself restore you and make you strong, firm and steadfast" (1 Peter 5:10). Someone once said it like this. When it comes to pain, God doesn't always give us answers, and He doesn't just give us advice. *But He does give us Himself.* The God of all grace will *Himself* restore us and make us strong, firm, and steadfast.

He was born in Wadowice, Poland, in 1920 and given the name Karol Józef Wojtyla.[9] His mother died when he was just nine; his brother, whom Karol adored, died when he was twelve.

He moved with his father to Krakow in 1938 and enrolled in the local university, where he showed great promise. He was especially adept at languages, eventually becoming fluent in twelve of them. But then evil intervened when Nazi Germany invaded Poland on September 1, 1939. The Nazis closed the university and required all students to perform manual labor; for the next few years, Karol worked in both a limestone quarry and a chemical factory—and his father died during that period.

It was while the Nazis controlled Poland that Karol felt the strong call of God on his life and determined he would become a priest. He enrolled in an underground seminary in Krakow. When the Nazis began to imprison all young Polish men to prevent an uprising, Karol hid himself in his uncle's basement. During those years, many of Karol's friends and fellow students were killed by the Nazis; some were shot by the Gestapo for the crime of studying for the priesthood. Karol himself was run over by a German truck but survived. Eventually the Nazis were driven out of Poland, but evil came calling to Poland under another dictator—Joseph Stalin.[10]

But after he had "suffered a little while," the God of all grace restored Karol and made him "strong, firm and steadfast." Karol persisted in his studies, earned two doctorates, and, in 1958, became the youngest bishop in Poland. In 1963 he became the Archbishop of Krakow; in 1967 he was promoted to the Sacred College of Cardinals; and in 1978 he was elected the youngest Pope in history—renamed Pope John Paul II. He remained pope until his death in 2005.[11]

His years as pope were marked by two themes—suffering and faithfulness. He was shot in 1981 in St. Peter's Square when an extremist tried to assassinate him; he survived after a five-hour surgery. Famously, he personally visited his assailant in prison to tell him that he forgave him.[12] In 2001 Pope John Paul II was diagnosed with Parkinson's disease, which eventually contributed to his death. But through it all he remained faithful to his calling and to his God. In 1984 he wrote an Apostolic Letter on suffering titled *Salvifici Doloris,* in which he addressed suffering's causes and meaning. In some of his closing words he wrote this to his fellow sufferers: "In the terrible battle between the forces of good and evil, revealed to our eyes by our modern world, may your suffering in union with the Cross of Christ be victorious!"[13] Karol Józef Wojtyla was both witness to and the victim of much evil in his life and suffered great pain because of it. But the God of all grace gave him the strength he needed to live, to serve, and to lead well.

But here's the next question—how does God's grace help us, practically and specifically, when the pain persists? And how does God's grace enable us to live with our pain without becoming one? Let's keep going and see if we can discover how to make a place for grace.

"When pain wears me down:
Make a place for grace."

CHAPTER NINE

The game, my older brothers told me, is called "99." Actually, it was a game only to them; it certainly wasn't a game for me. They would pin my scrawny body to the ground and hold my arms by placing their knees on my elbows, and then they would proceed to administer ninety-nine light taps to my sternum. They weren't hard blows, mind you; I could not honestly complain that they were "hitting" me. They were just taps—one after another after another. But by the time the count got to about sixty or seventy, those taps began to take their toll. My bony little sternum got sorer and sorer. And by the time they got into the nineties, each tap felt like I was being slugged. One or two taps was no big deal. Thirty or forty taps, I could handle. But ninety-nine taps—that was misery.

And sometimes that's what pain does to us—*it just plain wears us down*. We can handle it for a while. After all, everybody hurts from time to time. You stub your toe; you hit your funny bone; you get a headache; your muscles get sore from working out. Or maybe the pain is more emotional than physical. You get turned down for a date. A friend says something that hurts your feelings.

Your family pet passes away and suddenly the house feels empty and quiet. But in time, you heal, or at least you learn to cope. You've heard the old adage that "time heals all wounds"? As some have pointed out, if that were entirely true, then we wouldn't need to actually see the doctor; we'd just have to sit in the waiting room.

But for the most part, we humans are pretty resilient. We've learned how to bounce back. We take our medicine; we get our therapy; we do what we need to do to get better. But that doesn't work if the source of the pain isn't removed, because each new day and each new night brings a new injury. Sometimes life pins us to the ground and plays "99" with us. The first blow isn't so bad, but it doesn't stop with just one. The next day there's another one, and the next day another one, and there's simply no opportunity to recover. I've never been in chemotherapy, but I have watched people go through that experience as they became physically and emotionally worn down by the relentlessness of their treatment.

My hunch is that you know what I'm talking about, that you've endured a season of life where the hits just kept coming. It's like being caught in a stormy sea where the waves continue to crash over you and push you down; you keep fighting to get your head above water to catch your breath, and as soon as you do, here comes another wave to pull you back under.

For the better part of two years, I could not get a break from the pain radiating from my hip to my foot and my back. I'd go to a doctor and he would ask me, "So when does it hurt? Is it when you get up from sitting down? Is it when you're going up stairs?" And I would say, "It always hurts." "Well, what about at night? How are you sleeping?" And I would say, "It always hurts." Fortunately, my wife would be there to support my story, because it sounds a little overblown, and she would explain to the doctor that even in my sleep I moaned and groaned and thrashed around.

There were two things I mainly used to help manage my pain. One was a product called Biofreeze. It comes either as a gel or a spray, and it does pretty much what the name implies—it freezes the part of the body you spray it on. The downside of Biofreeze is that it smells. After spraying Biofreeze all over my back, I smelled like a walking locker room. The second way I handled my pain was with ice packs. I sat with ice on my back and had it on my leg during the day; I went to bed lying on ice; and the first question Brenda would ask me every morning was, "How many ice packs do you need?" I used ice packs so much that I wore holes in them and they stained my clothes and sheets. My favorite people were people who had found a new-and-improved ice pack or an ice pack that lasted longer or an ice pack that covered more of my body. And if you're wondering whether I ever got cold, I can tell you that I was always cold and often shivering, especially after I lost over 20 pounds, but I didn't care because it helped me cope with the pain.

You may know exactly what I'm talking about; you may well be going through a similar experience right now. You know what it's like when pain wears you down; you know the desperation. It's not that you want to die. More than anything you want to live; you'd love to have your life back. But you don't want to live like "this"— watching other people do what you can't . . . checking the clock to see if it's time to take your next pain pill . . . getting angry with your spouse for suggesting you look like you're better today when

you don't want to look better because you certainly don't feel better.

It was during those particularly rough days that my good friend Andrew, the worship leader for our church, shared the song "Worn" with me. It was by a group called Tenth Avenue North from their 2012 album called *The Struggle*. I knew of the group but had never heard of the song. He emailed me a link to the song and, while I am technologically challenged, I do know how to click on a link, so I began listening "I'm tired, I'm worn," the song begins, "from the work it takes to keep on breathing."[1] It went on, the writer describing a heavy heart, a crushed soul, and an ache for the pain to somehow come to an end. I listened, and I listened again, and I listened again. And the thought came to me—someone, somehow, wrote a song about me.

I'm pretty sure Andrew knew, when he sent me that song, that it was going to make me cry . . . which it did. But I treasured that song as a tremendously gracious and kind gift, because what it helped me feel was this very important truth—*somebody understands what my life feels like.* Somebody understands what it feels like when pain wears you down, when it feels like there's no hope, no way out, nothing to be done, no more options to try. Someone behind that song understood. And I knew this—Andrew understood. His pain and his wife Natalie's pain was and is a different kind of pain (the pain of childlessness) but it's a pain every bit as deep and unrelenting as the physical pain others of us have gone through.

So how do you handle pain when it wears you down? How do you live with such pain without becoming a pain? Here's my thought: *when pain wears you down, you have to make a place for grace.* Let me see if I can explain what I mean by that and how to do it, how to make a place in your pain for grace.

GOD'S PROMISE—
MY GRACE IS SUFFICIENT

First, let's remind ourselves of a promise God made to us through the pen of the Apostle Paul—*God promised us that His grace would be sufficient.* By way of reminder, of the twenty-seven books of the New Testament, Paul wrote thirteen of them. He is rightly regarded as the greatest missionary of all time. But while Paul had a great deal of success as a missionary and a writer, he suffered tremendously. And just as every one of us would do, Paul got on his knees and pleaded with God to take away his pain. Listen to what Paul writes about a conversation he had with God regarding a certain hardship that just wouldn't go away, what Paul refers to as a "thorn in the flesh":

> To keep me from becoming conceited because of these surpassingly great revelations, there was given me a thorn in my flesh, a messenger of Satan, to torment me. Three times I pleaded with the Lord to take it away from me. But he said to me, "My grace is sufficient for you, for my power is made perfect in weakness." Therefore I will boast all the more gladly about my weaknesses, so that Christ's power may rest on me. That is why, for Christ's sake, I delight in weaknesses, in insults, in hardships, in persecution, in difficulties. For when I am weak, then I am strong (2 Corinthians 12:7–10 niv84).

We don't know what Paul was referring to by the term "thorn in the flesh." Whatever it was, it was more than a hangnail. Paul says that Satan used this thorn to "torment" him. Has there ever been anything in your life so bad, so hard, so painful, that you could say it tormented or haunted or plagued you? Maybe it's a memory that haunts you, a memory of something that went terribly wrong or a memory of something you did terribly wrong. Maybe it's a physical ailment that makes it painful to stand, sit, or sleep—my brother's back pain is like that. Maybe it's something you *don't* have, an emptiness that at times is consuming. Maybe it's the pain of loneliness. (A research study at UCLA in 2003 discovered that loneliness actually triggers activity in some of the same regions of the brain that register physical pain.[2]) And maybe, like Paul, you have begged God over and over to do something, to put an end to the torment, to relieve the pain, to fill the void, to heal the memory, to remove the thorn . . . and so far, God hasn't done it.

But notice God's answer to Paul's prayer. Our usual response when God doesn't do for us what we asked Him to is complain about God's lack of concern or doubt that God is even there. But just because God doesn't do what we asked Him to doesn't mean that He isn't there or that He doesn't care or that He's unfair. God always hears our prayers, but sometimes—perhaps often—His answer to us is the same answer He gave to Paul: "My grace is sufficient for you."

Let's think about that word *sufficient* for a minute. God told Paul that His grace was sufficient, that it was ample, that His grace was everything Paul needed to live well even though he had a thorn in the flesh Satan was using to torment him. Now let's ask the question that's in the back of our minds anyway: is God just humoring Paul? Is this God's way of pacifying Paul, of getting Paul off His back? Think of it like this. Your daughter begs you over and over to buy her a car. You don't want to sound like a complete jerk and just tell her no, so you say to her, "Honey, I'm not going to give you a car, but I want you to know how proud I am of you. I can't give you what you asked for, but I'll always give you what you really need. Here, let me give you a hug." Is that all God is saying to Paul? Is God saying, "Paul, I'm sorry, but I'm not able to help you with that thorn-in-the-flesh thing. But I do want you to know that I love you and I'm proud of you and I'm always here to listen. Now get lost and stop your whining."

No, that's not what God was saying to Paul. Here's what God was saying: "Paul, I'm sorry, but I'm not going to remove the thorn from your flesh. I know it's painful and that it makes your life much harder, but for reasons you wouldn't completely understand right now, it's better for you that I don't take it away. But, Paul, listen to me carefully. *I am going to give you everything you need to live—and to live well—despite the thorn in your flesh.* Whatever you need to handle your pain, Paul, I can give you—courage, perspective, strength, stamina, energy . . . . My grace is everything you need."

I'm guessing you know someone who is the perfect example of God's sufficient grace, a person who is going through a very hard time and yet lives with an elegance of spirit that is captivating. Eloise is 89; she has, for years, suffered with terrible pain in her spine, legs, and feet. Her doctor gives her pain medicine to relieve it enough so she can get a few hours of sleep each night, but even so sleep is elusive. She should be tired and cranky all the time; she would have the right to complain all the time; she would be forgiven for expecting people to care for her all the time—she's 89 and in pain, after all. But Eloise still lives in her own home, still drives, still cares largely for herself, and is the life of the party every Sunday night when the extended family gathers for dinner. Her faith is infectious, her joy contagious. You would think she would be worn down by her pain and, well—at 89—by life. But Eloise would tell you this: God's grace is sufficient.

So that's God's promise to all of us who have been worn down by pain—God promises to give us all the grace we need. *He promises to give us the power to live well even though the thorn is still poking us in the flesh.* We'll come back to how that works practically in a moment, but for now let's acknowledge that God does promise to provide us with grace to handle the pain that refuses to leave us alone.

GOD'S OFFER— MY COMPASSIONS ARE NEW EVERY MORNING

So that's God's promise; let me show you something else God offers us. This is a passage and a truth my grandmother taught me many years ago. I was twenty, and my dad had just died at the age of fifty-four from a heart attack, an event which significantly changed my mom's life and my life (being the only one of the three boys who still had responsibilities at home). Nanny, as we called her, loved to sing hymns, although she was completely tone deaf . . . painfully tone deaf. One of her favorite hymns was called "Great Is Thy Faithfulness," and as she and I were talking about my dad's passing, she took out her well-worn Bible to show me where the lyrics of "Great Is Thy Faithfulness" come from. It's in a book in the Old Testament called Lamentations. A "lament" is a passionate expression of grief; Lamentations is really a book of tears. For most of the book's five chapters, the author—likely the prophet Jeremiah—complains about how God has made his life and the lives of his people miserable. Listen to how this devout servant of God talks to and about God: "He has driven me away and made me walk in darkness rather than light; . . . He has made my skin and my flesh grow old and has broken my bones. He has besieged me and surrounded me with bitterness and hardship. . . . Even when I call out or cry for help, he shuts out my prayer" (Lamentations 3:2, 4–5, 8).

"Nanny," I said, "why are you reading this to me? It sure doesn't sound very encouraging." Then Nanny dramatically turned the page of her Bible and took us to some verses just a little bit later in Lamentations 3. She then read me these words: "Yet this I call to mind and therefore I have hope: Because of the LORD's great love we are not consumed, for his compassions never fail. They are new every morning; great is your faithfulness. I say to myself, 'The LORD is my portion; therefore I will wait for him.'" (Lamentations 3:21–24).

Here's God's offer to us—He offers a fresh dose of his love and grace every morning. When our kids were much younger, I would often be the one in charge of getting them breakfast. One of them would come to me and say, "I'm hungry," and my usual response to them was this: "How can you be hungry? We just fed you yesterday!" I think they might have laughed once or twice—you know, the "polite" laugh. But usually they just ignored me because they knew that every morning they would be provided breakfast. True, it was usually a Pop Tart or some days a "Lego" frozen waffle or Frosted Flakes (I hope my wife isn't reading this). But they knew that even though they had eaten the day before, they were still going to be offered something new to eat when the morning came.

Yesterday may have been a hard one for you; it may have been a day of pain, pain that wore you down. You survived it. God's grace was sufficient for the day—He gave you a healthy perspective on your pain and your life; He gave you the resolve to soldier through another day; He brought someone into your life who helped you laugh. But then you woke up today and your first thought was, "I still hurt." And you wondered, "How am I going to do this again? How am I going to get through another day?"

At least that's what I think most mornings when I wake up. I wake up most every morning in pain. That specific pain doesn't usually last all that long, but it's how I begin every day. And I'll be honest—I don't always wake up particularly happy. I often wake up just a little bit depressed. And many mornings, this passage comes to mind, the one my grandmother taught me: "His compassions never fail; they are new every morning." It comes to mind even when I don't want it to, even when I would prefer to sit and moan and complain.

But here's the question: how do we receive God's love and His grace? God promises that His grace will be sufficient, that it's everything we need to live well even when we're still in pain. And He offers to give us a fresh dose of it every morning. God never says to us, "How can you need more grace? I gave you grace yesterday!" His compassions are new every morning. But you and I both know that the experience of God's grace is not automatic. He doesn't force it on us. He doesn't compel us to eat the fresh breakfast He's prepared for us. There is still our part, our role, our responsibility.

Our Role—
Make a Place for God's Grace

And here's what our role is—*to make a place for God's grace.* We need to make room in our hearts and in our lives for God to move in so He can give us His healing, empowering, all-sufficient grace.

Do you have a favorite place? It's probably somewhere in your home, the place where you feel the most comfortable and secure. Mine is on my couch in the family room. My place has a recliner and a cup holder and is perfectly situated in front of the TV. It's kind of like Sheldon's spot in *The Big Bang Theory.* I have a place for my remote, a place for my Diet Pepsi, a place for my iPad, a place for my phone, and a place for my magazines and books. So if my wife wants to sit close to me, I have to make a place for her.

But when Brenda comes to sit by me, I know she doesn't simply want me to clear some space so she can sit down. She wants me to make a place for her in my heart. And if you've been worn down by pain, you know that takes a conscious effort. One of the things that makes a person in pain a pain to be around is that we sometimes simply refuse to let people in. We pull the hoodie up over our head and pretend to listen to their words of encouragement, but we make it pretty clear that we just don't have room for them right now. It's a foolish thing to do. It's a selfish thing to do, and we know it. But sometimes we choose to do it anyway—we choose not to make room for them.

And just like we do that to the people who love us, we do it to God. We shut Him out. Sometimes we shut out God because we're a little ticked off that He's allowed this to happen to us. But sometimes we do it because it's too hard to engage, like it's too much effort to make room for God. What I think happens to us some-times when pain wears us down is that we get passive. Everything feels so hard that we sort of shut down, physically and emotionally and spiritually. It's like when you don't use your computer for a while and it goes into "sleep mode" to conserve energy. We sort of do that; we sort of just shut down to conserve energy and protect our hurting hearts.

But every morning God comes to us and says, "I've got some-thing for you; I've got just what you need to live well today even while the pain persists." And what we have to do is to consciously choose to receive God's grace. We need to make a place in our hearts and our lives for God's grace to work.

I've told you about my place on my favorite couch. Mornings are still a challenge for me, so what I do most mornings is to sit in my place. I usually have a Pop Tart—the breakfast of champions. I often watch a little bit of the *Today Show*. But mostly I just sit there. I used to sit there when I was at my worst and tell myself "I'll never get better." It's embarrassing to tell you that, but I'm afraid it's true. But now I'm telling myself something different, what my grandmother taught me forty years ago. Let me show you the verses again: "Yet this I call to mind and therefore I have hope: Because of the LORD's great love we are not consumed, for his compas-sions never fail. They are new every morning; great is your faithful-ness. I say to myself, 'The LORD is my portion; therefore I will wait for him'" (Lamentations 3:21–24). The last sentence is what my grandmother taught me to say. So I sit there and I wait. I mentally make a place on my couch for God to come meet me and give me the grace I need for the day. There were some days when that took quite a while. More recently the wait has gotten shorter. But He has always come, He has always gotten me up off the couch, and He has always given me what I needed for the day.

There are other things I do now to make a place for grace in my life, too, and I imagine they're not much different from what you do. I listen to hopeful music. And when I get to my office, I pull out my Bible and spend some time listening to the Spirit of God. One of the most important ways for us to make a place for grace is to make a place for people, to not only engage with people when they come to us but to take the initiative and go to them. One way or another, we need to give God room to work, to make a place in our lives where He can pour His grace into us and shower us with His compassions. Maybe your place for grace is a coffee shop where you start your mornings—having your favorite morning drink, listening to music, watching people around you come to life, and inviting God to work in your heart to bring you to life. Maybe your place for grace is at gym. The gym? I know, there's not much you can do, and so many others can do so much more. But you can do something—your therapist showed you what she wants you to do. You could find your place on the mat, do the stretches you're supposed to do, breathe . . . and wait for God to open up your heart to the gift of a new day.

And when we make a place for grace, here's what we will discover; I've begun to discover it myself. In the words of the song "Worn," we'll discover that "redemption wins, that the struggle ends, that God can mend a heart that's frail and torn. We'll discover that a song can rise from the ashes of a broken life and all that's dead inside can be reborn."[3]

Pain can wear you down. But here's the good news: in the end, grace wins.

**"When my pain is their gain:
How not to waste a hurt."**

CHAPTER TEN

Because my grandparents and parents lived through the Great Depression way back in the 1930s, we kids were taught from an early age that it was a sin to waste anything. The opening of presents on Christmas Eve became something of a marathon in our family because my grandmother insisted we not tear the wrapping paper, as that would be wasteful. Instead, we had to use scissors to carefully cut the tape and then slowly unwrap the present and give the paper to Nanny so she could neatly fold it up and save it for next year.

My grandfather was just as careful about not wasting anything. He never used Kleenex because it bothered him to throw the Kleenex away after blowing his nose. Instead, he used handkerchiefs, which could be washed and used over and over. And while I never went to some of those extremes, I have to admit that some of their values rubbed off on me. When we were first married and had very little in the way of income, I was very careful about conserving energy. I grew up in Minnesota, where the winters can be a bit cold, so I felt it was wasteful to set our thermostat above 60 degrees during the day—and it was a real waste to have the heat on at all at night. Brenda (a California girl) and I had a few discussions about that, as you can guess. And she will be glad to tell you about the many winter nights when we were first married and wore hooded sweatshirts to bed to keep our ears warm. I will have to admit, it was not very romantic.

You may not have grown up in the Great Depression, but no matter what age you are, you've been taught not to waste valuable resources. When I was a kid, there were a fair number of things we just threw away. But not anymore—we recycle. We recycle paper to the extent that we don't even print things anymore. We recycle soda cans and water bottles, cardboard boxes, grass clippings, and yard waste. We used to recycle grocery bags, but we decided that was wasteful, so now we bring our own bags to the grocery store so we can reuse them.

And just as we don't want to waste energy or paper or bottles or cans, we surely don't want to waste our hurts. Now, I understand that we all want to move past our pain. We don't want to reopen our wounds; we don't want to relive our injuries. We want nothing more than to put our pain in the rearview mirror. But many fellow sufferers who have gone before us have taught us a valuable lesson, and that is this: *never waste a hurt.*

Many of us remember when we heard the news of Rick and Kay Warren's son Matthew committing suicide. It was a horrible tragedy, a moment of untold pain and grief. Rick and Kay talked about it on national TV on *Piers Morgan Live* on CNN,[1] and Brenda and I had a chance to hear Rick talk about the experience in person less than a year after the event. He was obviously still grieving the death of his son; Rick said that he and Kay had cried over the loss of their son every day. But his talk to us had this title: "Never Waste Your Pain." What follows is part of what he shared with us that day, a talk I'll never forget.

Pastor Rick loves to use alliterative outlines, and this talk was no different. In *Sesame Street* terms, it was sponsored by the letter "S." Many of us are aware of the work of author Elisabeth Kubler-Ross who outlined the five stages of grief in her 1969 book *On Death and Dying*. I would guess many of us could even recite the five stages of grief: *denial, anger, bargaining, depression,* and, finally, *acceptance.* But Rick suggested a different way to look at the stages of grief that made a great deal of sense to me. See if they resonate at all with you.

First, Rick said, there's *shock*. Rick and Kay knew from the time Matthew was very young that he had mental health issues. Matthew talked with them often about suicide. They went with Matthew to specialists all around the country to get him help. So in one way, his suicide wasn't a surprise. But you and I know that every death is shocking, even if someone dies after a long illness. It takes your breath away; it disorients you. Or if you've been told you have a serious illness or a loved one is in an accident or you discover your partner has been unfaithful to you, you know how shock can wash over you and stop you in your tracks.

Second, Rick said, there's *sorrow*. And as Rick was quick to point out, sorrow is a godly emotion. It's not a sin to feel sorrow over death or disease or divorce. Jesus was, the Bible tells us, a "man of sorrows" (Isaiah 53:3 KJV). In 2 Corinthians 7, the Bible talks about what it calls "godly sorrow." God gave us the capacity to cry for a reason. Sorrow is an appropriate response to pain and loss.

Third, Rick said, there's *struggle*. We've said quite a lot about that so far. We've said it's okay to complain to God about our pain and our suffering, just as Job did, just as Jeremiah did in the book of Lamentations, just as many other men and women of God through the years have done. We struggle to make sense of our suffering. We struggle to understand why it's happening to us. We struggle to get our bearings, to regain our equilibrium. In the process, we might break a dish or two; we might say some things we never thought we'd say. The struggle is often exhausting. It can feel as if it's never going to end. And so we do our best to hang on.

Fourth, Rick said, there's *surrender*. This is where we who follow Jesus say to our God, "I don't understand this. I'm not happy about this. I would never choose this. But I trust You. I believe that You are good and almighty and loving and wise—and I believe that even though I can't see it, somehow and some way, You're going to use this for something good." This isn't giving up. It's not quitting. It's a choice; it's a decision to surrender your life to God, to put your life and your pain in His hands and to trust Him to see you through. Job said it this way: "Though [God] slay me, yet will I hope in him" (Job 13:15).

Fifth, Rick said, there's *sanctification*. Admittedly, this is a theological word. Piers Morgan looked a bit puzzled by this word, and I imagine many of those listening that day had never heard the word before. But you might remember what the Bible means by sanctification, which is the process of becoming more like Jesus. It means to grow spiritually, to grow in our character. It's when God begins to use our pain for our gain, when He uses our hurts to help us become more patient, more compassionate, to gain a healthier perspective about what really matters. This is what James is talking about when he writes this: "Consider it pure joy, my brothers and sisters, whenever you face trials of many kinds, because you know that the testing of your faith produces perseverance" (James 1:2–3). That's sanctification, when God uses our pain to help us grow in godliness.

And sixth, Rick said, there's *service*. By service, of course, Rick means that we reach the stage where we can use our pain to serve other people. That's what we mean when we say we're not to waste a hurt. But here's the reality—it's not natural, and it's not easy. Yet it's precisely what we as followers of Jesus have been called to do. We are called to serve out of our suffering. And it is a critical stage in learning to live with pain without becoming one.

Jesus—
the Suffering Servant

Shock, sorrow, struggle, surrender, sanctification, and service. Let's come at this point about service from a different angle for a moment and remind ourselves what God's larger goal is for our lives: it is that we become like Jesus in our character. Here's how the Living Bible puts it in the book of Romans: "For from the very beginning God decided that those who came to him—and all along he knew who would—should become like his Son, so that his Son would be the First, with many brothers" (Romans 8:29 TLB). One of Max Lucado's books is all about this subject; it's called quite simply *Just Like Jesus*.[2] That's God's goal for you and me, that as Christ's followers we become just like Him in the way we live our lives.

So then the question is, "How did Jesus live His life? What was He like?" Now there are lots of ways to describe how Jesus lived, so let's just focus on one most germane to this topic. One of Jesus's many titles in the Bible is this, the *Suffering Servant*. It comes from a series of four songs in the Old Testament book of Isaiah that predict the coming of the Messiah to save the people of God, and in those songs God's Servant is described as one who suffers. Jesus even applied these passages to Himself. On the road to Emmaus on the afternoon of His resurrection, Jesus told two of His followers, "Did not the Messiah have to suffer these things and then enter his glory?" (Luke 24:26).

The most famous description of the Suffering Servant is in Isaiah 53. You've likely heard some of these verses before: "He was despised and rejected by mankind, a man of suffering, and familiar with pain. Like one from whom people hide their faces he was despised, and we held him in low esteem. Surely he took up our pain and bore our suffering, yet we considered him punished by God, stricken by him, and afflicted. But he was pierced for our transgressions, he was crushed for our iniquities; the punishment that brought us peace was on him, and by his wounds we are healed" (Isaiah 53:3–5). The Jesus we follow is One who is familiar with pain and suffering. And notice *why* He suffered: it was for our benefit. He was pierced for our transgressions, crushed for our iniquities. He suffered to serve us and to save us.

A few chapters back, we talked about when pain is a calling and about the fact that sometimes it is God's will and plan for our lives that we suffer. This chapter again reminds us of that truth. Look at what Isaiah writes just a few verses later: "Yet it was the LORD's will to crush him and cause him to suffer" (Isaiah 53:10). Jesus's suffering was not an accident or a fluke of circumstances; it was by divine design. And the purpose of Jesus's suffering was to save us and serve us. Jesus said it Himself to His disciples: "Whoever wants to become great among you must be your servant, and whoever wants to be first must be your slave—just as the Son of Man did not come to be served, but to serve, and to give his life as a ransom for many" (Matthew 20:26–28). That is the Jesus we are called to follow. That is the Jesus we are to model ourselves after—Jesus, the Suffering Servant.

JESUS'S FOLLOWERS—
SUFFERING SERVANTS

In other words, we who follow Jesus should also be suffering servants. Certainly our suffering isn't the same as what Jesus suffered, and we can't possibly accomplish what He did through His suffering. But the principle is the same: we are called as Christ-followers to use our suffering and pain to serve other people.

Let me show you a passage that puts this very clearly for us, and then I'll try to be as practical as I can about how to do it. This is written by Paul, a suffering servant himself, in a letter to the church at Corinth:

> Praise be to the God and Father of our Lord Jesus Christ, the Father of compassion and the God of all comfort, who comforts us in all our troubles, so that we can comfort those in any trouble with the comfort we ourselves receive from God. For just as we share abundantly in the sufferings of Christ, so also our comfort abounds through Christ. If we are distressed, it is for your comfort and salvation; if we are comforted, it is for your comfort, which produces in you patient endurance of the same sufferings we suffer. (2 Corinthians 1:3–6)

If you've studied much grammar in your life or if you've ever studied a foreign language, you've probably heard of something called "the purpose clause." In this passage, those two words "so that" tell us it's part of a purpose clause. What's God's purpose in giving us comfort in our troubles? He comforts us *"so that"* we can comfort those in any trouble with the same comfort God gave us.

When you think about it, that's probably the main question we all have when we go through a period of pain—*what's the purpose of this?* What's the point? Why is this happening to me? I'm not going to tell you this is the whole answer; it's not. But here is part of the answer to that question, no matter what you're suffering through right now. *Part of the purpose of your pain is to prepare and equip you to help someone else through their pain.*

At the end of Rick Warren's talk that day on how not to waste a hurt, he told us to do this: "Write down the names of all the people you know who are going through something similar to what you've gone through." Notice he didn't say to write down the names of everyone who hurts . . . because that's everyone. But write down the names of people who have hurt in a similar way to the way you hurt. Why? Because those are the people you are best equipped to help. If you've lost a loved one in a drunk-driving accident, then the people who you are going to be able to comfort and encourage better than anyone else are people who've lost a loved one in a drunk-driving accident. If you've ever been diagnosed with cancer or had to go through chemo, you are far better equipped than me to minister to people who are battling cancer.

And let me suggest something. Don't wait until you're fully recovered before you start serving. Don't wait until the pain is gone before you reach out to other people in pain. And I say that for at least a couple of reasons. For one, when I was at my worst, I found that I received greater comfort from people who themselves were still in pain than I did with people who said, "Yeah, I went through something similar twenty years ago." Now, that person was still helpful; I needed to hear from someone who survived and got better. But the people whose comfort meant the most to me were the people who looked me in the eyes and said, "I am in pain all the time." And I didn't need those folk to say a whole lot to me. Just the fact that they made the effort to share a little of their story with me and hold my hand for a minute and tell me they would pray for me was incredibly comforting.

And here's another reason I encourage you to reach out even while the pain is fresh; let me give you an example. When I was twenty-two, I proposed to my girlfriend on Christmas Eve. I told my family and friends I was going to propose because I was so sure she was going to say yes. She didn't; she told me no. It was pretty humiliating. And for several years I could very much relate to people who were hurting because they had been rejected in one way or another. But that was decades ago. I've been married for over thirty-six years. Now I look back and I am incredibly grateful that she said no. So while I *remember* what it's like to be rejected, I don't *feel* it the same way anymore. So don't wait until your hurt is fully healed to use your experience to offer help to others. Just share where you are and anything you've learned about how to handle your particular brand of pain. What you have to say is likely to be far more helpful to your friend than anything they could read on the Internet.

Now maybe you're thinking, "Gee, I don't know anyone off the top of my head who I can help. I don't know anyone who is going through what I've gone through." My guess is that if you ask around just a little bit, if you share some of your story, you'll find plenty of folk very much like you. Or look up support groups for people who are facing your struggle—you'll definitely benefit from hearing their stories but, just as importantly, they need to hear yours. It might seem as if everyone around you is okay, but give people a chance to talk a little, to share some of their story, and you'll discover, like the old song says, that everybody hurts.

You've probably discovered some websites that offer both support for your struggle with pain and a place to help others. For example, the U.S. Pain Foundation has a website that offers numerous resources both for those dealing with pain and those who care for them.[3] Among the programs offered are "Take Control of Your Pain," which provides patient-education days for "pain warriors" and "care champions" to learn tools empowering them to take control of their pain and medical journeys; "Heroes of Healing," an online, closed support group that offers an opportunity for those in pain to connect in a safe, secure space; and "Pain Medicine 411," which provides information on the risks and benefits of prescription drugs.[4]

I read a helpful article by a young woman and gifted writer named Catherine Woodiwiss, who went through a series of traumas in a short period of time, including being hit by a car while biking and having to undergo one surgery after another. For quite a while she breathed and ate through a tube, unable to speak. And while she was still in the process of recovery, she wrote down some of what she'd learned about how to help people in pain. Here are a couple of the lessons she shared that particularly resonated with me.[5]

First, *do be there, but don't compare.* Some of us have been told that suffering people need their space, that they need to be left alone so they can sort things out. But most people in pain want and need company. As we've said before, no one should suffer alone. And Catherine makes an interesting point, saying it's much easier for a person in pain to say to a visitor, "Thanks for coming, but I need to be alone for a little bit," than it is to say, "I was in pain and nobody cared." When I had my first hip-replacement surgery, I really appreciated that people stopped by to let me know they hadn't forgotten me. And when I needed them to go, I learned that all I had to do was to say, "I think I'm going to throw up." Then they left very quickly. But err on the side of showing up and being present, and then pay attention to the cues the person you're visiting gives you.

So do be there, but *don't compare.* It's so tempting for us to say to the person in pain, "I know how you feel," because we do know how it feels to be in pain. But we *don't* know how *they* feel. Even when we've been through a very similar experience, we don't know how they feel. Let them tell you instead. Let them share their story, and then simply tell them you're so sorry.

Now, I know I'm mostly talking about how to be a comfort to those in pain, but let me say something to those who are being comforted. This goes in the column of how to live with pain without becoming a pain to those who care about you. If someone tells you they know how you feel—when you know they really don't—do your best to accept their condolences with grace. In other words, don't be a jerk about it. First Corinthians 13 is known to Bible students as the "love chapter," and I really like how the Living Bible translates verse 7 where it says that love always believes in him and always expects the best of him. If someone takes the time to visit you but says something that's not very helpful, believe the best about that person; trust that they're trying to be helpful and it just came out wrong. If you've just suffered a horrible trauma and someone says, "I know how you feel; I had to take my dog to the vet last week," just say, "Thank you for caring" . . . and then tell them you think you have to throw up.

Here's another insight Catherine Woodiwiss shares: *a person in pain needs two different kinds of helpers—the firefighter and the builder.* The firefighter is the kind of person who will drop whatever they're doing and rush to the scene to help the sufferer. This is the person who sits with you in the hospital, who brings you a meal every day for a week, who goes to the store to pick up your prescriptions, and who does all those things for you that you can't do in the first days of your pain. That person is a treasure, a true hero. But just as heroic is the person Catherine calls the builder. This is the person who helps you do whatever it takes to rebuild your life. This is a long-term position. This is a job that takes weeks and months and often years. And here's a very helpful insight Catherine makes: *very few people can be both the firefighter and the builder.* Most people are wired to be one kind of caregiver or the other. So don't hold it against your spouse or your friends if they aren't good at both roles, because pretty much none of us are. Don't be angry if the person who was there for you every minute of Days 1 through 7 doesn't show up as much anymore. And don't be angry that the person who is taking you to rehab twice every week for a year wasn't there with you every second in the hospital when you first got hurt.

For you who are caregivers—and that should be all of us at one time or another—don't feel guilty that you can't be everything the person in pain needs. Give what you have to give; care out of your own wounded heart as best you can. Be the best firefighter you can be; be the best builder you can be. But realize that you alone can never do it all, and you can never be all that the person in pain needs. Take them to the Person who *can* be all the person in pain needs—take them to Jesus. Don't be afraid to ask your friend, "Can I pray for you right now?" Help your friend connect to the Suffering Servant Himself, the one Person who really does know how they feel and who can heal the hurts no human doctor can.

WHEN YOU'VE TRIED EVERYTHING
AND NOTHING WORKS

We've covered a lot, and I imagine you've tried a lot to help you with your pain. So my next question is, what do you do when you've tried everything and you still hurt and it feels like you've run out of options? Is there anything more to do when you've flat-out done it all?

"When you've tried everything:
Do healthy things."

CHAPTER ELEVEN

So you've tried everything you know to manage your pain and it still hurts and you're no less frustrated. By the way, it turns out there's quite a lot to try. The U.S. Pain Foundation lists forty-six different "complementary therapies" that "have the potential to lower our pain or help us find balance and stability in the midst of chaos and pain."[1] Some of them are pretty mainstream: active-release technique, chiropractic, massage therapy, and music therapy, to name a few. Others seem a bit of a stretch, like crystal therapy, for example. Here's part of the description: "These precious stones pass their healing powers on to others through the etheric energy field that surrounds the body. Crystals have the ability to cure all ailments and bring peace and tranquility into one's life."[2] This organization offers pain warriors loads of helpful resources, but this particular claim seems to promise more than it can deliver. Crystals can cure all ailments? Maybe I'm too skeptical, but I just don't buy it.

And that's not all. Some studies suggest that virtual reality can offer at least temporary relief to people who suffer from chronic pain. Then there's "aura imaging," "Bach flowers," "chakra alignment," "colonics" (and, yes, that's about cleaning out your colon), "feng shui," "magnets," "Reiki," and more. To be honest, I didn't try any of those—I'm not quite sure I would know how. But I did try a fair number of complementary therapies, including active-release technique, myofascial massage, chiropractic work, exercise, and heat therapy. Did they help? The myofascial massage does help to some degree; I have a terrific therapist. But the reality is that no matter what I do, the pain is still there . . . every day and every night.

So why keep trying? What's the point? If there's nothing I can do to eliminate my pain, then why bother making the effort?

Because I need to. I need to for the sake of my soul, and I need to for the sake of the people who love me. And because God tells me to.

The verse isn't strictly on-point; Paul didn't write this with chronic-pain sufferers in mind. But I think it fits; I think it's part of what God is telling me about how to live with pain without becoming one: "Let us not become weary in doing good, for at the proper time we will reap a harvest if we do not give up" (Galatians 6:9).

Keep doing good. Don't give up. Even if the pain doesn't go away.

Chester W. Nimitz was an admiral who played a significant role in World War II as commander in chief of the United States Pacific Fleet. One of the main highways I often drive in Northern California is named in his honor—the Nimitz Freeway. But it's a prayer he prayed that has most impacted me, a simple prayer I've learned to make my own: "God, grant me the courage not to give up what I think is right, even though I think it hopeless."

Have you ever heard of the "Anyway" poem? It's often attributed to Mother Teresa, in part because it was found posted on the wall of Mother Teresa's home for children in Calcutta, India, but it was originally written by Dr. Kent M. Keith (when he was a nineteen-year-old sophomore at Harvard) and titled "The Paradoxical Commandments." Here's an excerpt: "If you do good, people will accuse you of selfish, ulterior motives. Do good anyway. . . . The good you do today will be forgotten tomorrow. Do good anyway. . . ."[3]

There are certain things that are good and right and healthy for us to do. Under normal circumstances, doing those things would ameliorate the pain and make us feel better. But not anymore. And yet we do them . . . anyway. Why? Because they are good and right and healthy.

AN EXAMPLE: EXERCISE . . . ANYWAY

Let me give you an example, to make this a bit more practical. Every caregiver and medical professional tells us that we need to exercise, that even if it exacerbates our pain, exercise is good for our overall well-being. I've never been fond of exercising for the sake of exercise. I preferred getting my exercise recreationally. For example, I wasn't fond of running for running's sake, but I loved to run if I could chase a ball—a tennis ball, a baseball, a football, or, preferably, a basketball. But given the poor outcome of my hip replacement, those sports are off the table. (Okay, I'm also getting a little old to play certain sports, but I'd rather blame my health than my age.) Basketball, my favorite activity, is simply too painful and too hard on my hip. I can't run, not even to get out of the way of a car. But I can do a variety of cardio exercises at the gym—the elliptical machines and various bikes work just fine for me.

But here's the thing. I don't like to use them. They're boring. No ball is involved. There's nothing fun about them. And when I'm done, I hurt all the more.

But I exercise . . . anyway.

So does Ryan. I met Ryan years ago at the gym where I've long been a member. Ryan is many years my junior, but we ran into each other enough that we became casual friends. Then Ryan stopped coming to the gym. I didn't have his number, so I couldn't call him, but after asking around, I learned that Ryan had been in an accident on his motorcycle—a serious accident. Months later I was working on the bench press when, out of the corner of my eye, I saw someone who reminded me of Ryan. His hair was much longer and he had a tattoo, but the biggest difference was his leg. It was different—it was titanium. And he *was* Ryan. I caught up to him and asked him how he was doing. It had been an ordeal, he explained. He crashed his motorcycle going over 65 mph and had lost a great deal of blood. His arm was damaged, and his leg—well, I could see what had happened to his leg.

Ryan is doing well now. He's walking with God, he's married and has a family, and he has a great job. And he's at the gym almost every day, working out as hard as anyone there, even though no amount of exercise is going to restore his leg. And while Ryan never complains, I know his workouts have a tendency to increase his pain. But he does it . . . anyway. He exercises because he knows it's good and right and healthy. It might not make his leg feel better, but it's good for his heart and his lungs and his brain.

And it's good for his soul. To keep doing those things we know are good and right and healthy enrich our souls even if they don't relieve our pain. And ultimately, a healthy soul is far more important to us than a body free of pain.

Here's how Jesus put it: "What good is it for someone to gain the whole world, yet forfeit their soul? Or what can anyone give in exchange for their soul?" (Mark 8:36–37). In his book *"Soul Keeping: Caring for the Most Important Part of You,"* John Ortberg explains it this way: "If your soul is healthy, no external circumstance can destroy your life. If your soul is unhealthy, no external circumstance can redeem your life."[4]

When I do things I know I should do—those things we all agree are good and right and healthy—it nourishes my soul. It especially nourishes my soul when I do those things "anyway," when I do them even though there's no payoff in the pain-relief department. When I quit doing what I know I should do, my soul is diminished. I feel weaker; I feel ashamed; I feel unworthy. But when I choose to do those things "anyway," my soul gets a little stronger. I feel more content, more at peace, more whole.

FROM THE CAREGIVER'S PERSPECTIVE

And let's not forget to look at this from the perspective of those who love us and are caring for us. They just want us to get better, and it pains them to see us continue to live in pain. But what pains them even more is to see us quit trying, to watch us give up.

After a joint replacement, the doctor sends you to physical therapy. Physical therapists seem to come in one of two sizes; it's either a diminutive young woman or an oversized, unshaved man. I chose the diminutive young woman, thinking she would surely be more sympathetic and gentle. I thought that if I groaned in pain she'd say, "There, there" and tell me I could quit. Not the case. Apparently physical therapy is only deemed effective if you groan. Let's just say the diminutive young female therapist made me do things I didn't like to do, and when I asked why I had to do them, she would simply say, "Because they're good for you." And the oversized, unshaved therapist working on the victim next to me simply nodded his head in agreement, just to make sure I got the message.

So I went to physical therapy for a few sessions. Didn't like it a bit. It was hard and I hurt worse when I was done, but the doctor and the therapist (and my wife) said it was good for me. Then one day I decided I wasn't going anymore. I didn't think it was helping me. I certainly didn't think it was worth the effort. And I thought my wife would be okay with this. After all, it meant one less thing she had to take me to, one less detour in her otherwise-hectic day. But she wasn't happy. She was . . . what's the word? . . . peeved. Probably not a strong enough word, but I think you get the idea. And, frankly, it wasn't that she was angry with me that bothered me the most; it's that she was disappointed in me.

And I got it, again. I had become a pain to the person who was giving 150 percent of herself to helping me get better. Brenda was working full-time along with taking care of the house and cooking the meals and caring for me, and I had one job—to work on getting better. And what was I doing? I was quitting. It was too hard and it didn't seem to be helping, so why try? And the answer to that question became obvious—for my wife. Sure, I needed to do it for me, for my soul. But I also needed to do it for her. Yes, she needed to hear me tell her "Thank you," but what she needed even more was to see me display the courage to do what was good and right and healthy "anyway," even if I didn't think it helped my pain. That was how I could honor her sacrifices and her devotion in a way that encouraged and respected her.

Maybe you're a son or daughter who is going to great lengths to encourage and care for your mom. She's been dealt an entirely unfair hand—she developed a debilitating illness and her husband left her rather than stay by her side. Her body betrayed her, and so did the one who promised to be there for her "in sickness and in health." So you do your best to step up and help your mom fight through her hardship and grief. You empathize, you console, you bring her groceries, you help her clean, you help manage her finances. And in return . . . you need to see her try. You can be the best son or daughter there could ever be for her, but you can't possibly be the only person in her life. You need to see her make the effort to reconnect with friends and family, with people who have cared for her over the years. You need to see her take the initiative to develop new relationships and find other sources of support. As the husband of a woman battling cancer told me, every so often it would encourage him to hear his wife ask someone *besides him* for help. He is absolutely devoted to her, but he knows he can't do it all for her, and it helps him to see her acknowledge that by making the effort to reach out to others herself.

HEALTHY THINGS
WE KNOW WE SHOULD DO

I'm guessing I don't have to tell you the things we should do anyway. But just to get the mental juices flowing a bit, let me make some suggestions.

Let's break them down into two larger categories—healthy

things, and the good and right things. First, the healthy things. We know we should exercise, so do whatever your doctor or therapist says you can and should do, and make it a habit. Then there's your diet. This isn't one of my favorites either. When you're in pain, it's pretty natural to justify a lousy diet by telling yourself, "I deserve this; I deserve to eat whatever I want, whenever I want, because it's the only thing that makes me feel better." But we know it's not healthy. We know we're only sabotaging ourselves. Eat healthy . . . anyway. I won't try to tell you what that is; that would be hypocritical. But you know, so do it. And if your doctor tells you to take vitamins and supplements, take those too.

Just a couple more. Clean yourself up. It's natural when the pain won't go away to get a bit lazy. Why? Because you deserve a break. So you don't shave, you don't change out of your favorite sweatpants, you don't brush your hair, and you don't pick up your room. Those things take too much effort when it takes everything in you just to do what you have to do. But it turns out people notice those things—things like how you smell. If you want to live with pain without becoming one, clean yourself up—shave, shower, pick up, wash your clothes. It's the healthy thing to do.

Last one. Get out of the house. Get out in the sun. Watch the birds soar overhead. Go to the mall. Yes, it's an effort and, yes, it will make you mad that most of the people you see appear to be moving without any pain while your pain level keeps rising, but you need to remind yourself that the world is bigger than your family room and there are more people in the world than the actors you watch on TV. Oh, and while you're out, make sure you find at least one thing that makes you laugh. Laughing is good for you, and seeing you laugh will make your caregiver's day.

And then there's the other category—the good and right things to do. Together we could make quite a long list, but let me suggest just three. For one, express appreciation and/or affection to someone every day. Certainly we need to thank those closest to us regularly; I'm sure my wife and friends never get tired of me telling them "Thank you." The Bible says this: "But encourage one another daily . . . (Hebrews 3:13). Thank your partner. Send a text to your friend to let them know you're praying for them. Forward an article to your buddy that you know he'd be interested in reading, just to let him know that what matters to him matters to you. Call your mom or your daughter; send a card to someone you miss seeing. And do it every day, even if people don't always respond, even if it's an effort, because it's a good and right thing to do, because God told us not to become weary in doing good.

Here's a second one in the "good and right" category: give. Yes, I'm talking about money. You already know this—managing your pain can be an expensive sport. Insurance can cover quite a bit, but it doesn't cover everything. There are doctors' bills, therapists' bills, pain medications . . . There are all those things you think are silly until you discover just how much you need them—the elevated toilet seat, the sock helper (not being able to put on your socks is a particularly humiliating experience when, in your head, you're still a high school athlete), the bath chair, the orthotics, and on it goes. And then there's the other kind of therapy that seems so necessary in managing your pain—retail therapy. Nothing else makes the pain go away, so maybe this will: more stuff! A new laptop or tablet or car! Just imagining having a bigger, brighter ultra HD TV in my family room (or wait . . . the bedroom!) is making me feel better.

But the good and right thing to do, and we know it, is to

give, to be generous. Give to your church. Sponsor a child through World Vision or Compassion International or Food for the Hungry and engage with that child by writing and sending pictures. Find a cause that strikes a chord in your heart and give to it, regularly, sacrificially. It's good and it's right and it will grow your soul.

Last suggestion—pray. I know, you're already praying. Every day you're talking to God, asking Him to take away the pain. Keep doing that. God loves the sound of your voice. But in addition to praying about your pain, pray about the needs of other people. If you're one of those whose pain has in one way or another put you on the sidelines and prevented you from doing all the things you used to do, you may well have more time to pray than some others do. The temptation is to use that time to escape. You know what I mean; we all do it. We escape through television, video games, fantasy novels, surfing the web . . . Some of that is fine. Jesus loved telling a good story, so there's no shame in reading or watching one. But God doesn't mean for us to escape life; He means for us to engage in it. And if our pain prevents us from engaging in life in some ways we did before, we can still engage in it in a significant way, and that's through prayer. James, in the Bible, says it like this: "The prayer of a righteous person is powerful and effective" (James 5:16). Maybe you can't do all the things for your partner that they can do for you, but you can make a difference in their life by pray-ing for them. Pray for your partner, your parents, your siblings, your children, your coworkers, your church, and your neighbors. Your pain may limit your enjoyment of your world, but it need not limit the impact you make on it.

Agnes was my great-aunt, the sister of my mom's mom; we called her Ann. Ann moved from Norway to Brooklyn to help my grandmother when my mom was born. My grandfather was, I am told, most appreciative of Ann's help, but he was a bit surprised that Ann ended up living with them for the rest of her life. Ann never married, and never—to my knowledge—had a job outside the home. She worked tirelessly at my grandparents' house and at her church; she was anything but lazy. But the thing she did the most, and best, was to pray. During the years I was growing up, Ann went to church every day. There weren't services every day, but that's where she went to pray.

The last few years of Ann's life were quite miserable for her. My grandparents, who were very poor, couldn't care for her physical needs and couldn't afford to pay for a private-care facility, so Ann went to the nursing home that Social Services said was her only choice. The staff there did their best, but the facilities were decidedly subpar. I was in my early twenties at the time, going to school and working two jobs, but I did my best to visit Ann whenever I could. Sometimes I would find Ann in her wheelchair, left out in the hallway, moaning in terrible pain. I would notify the nurses of her situation and ask them to get her something for her pain. Then I would get Ann's attention, hold her otherworldly soft hands, and wheel her to her room so we could talk and she could get away from the noise of the other residents. She would ask me how I was, and I would ask about her—what she was eating, who she talked to, what she did there. But I knew what she did. She couldn't see well enough to read; she couldn't watch TV. Actually, she wouldn't have done those things anyway, because she was too busy praying. She prayed for my grandparents. She prayed for her church. She prayed for my family. And she prayed for me.

Whatever I've accomplished in my life, whatever I have

become, I know this—I am who I am in part because of Ann's prayers. I know Ann asked God to take away her pain, because I prayed those prayers with her. God didn't. I know Ann asked God to get her out of the nursing home; God didn't. But Ann prayed . . . anyway. And because she did, scores of lives have been changed forever.

Good things, right things, healthy things—you do them and the pain doesn't go away. Do them anyway.

**"When pain meets its match:
There's hope for the long haul."**

CHAPTER TWELVE

I t's an old story now, the classic Charles Dickens story *A Christmas Carol*, but there's a scene from that story that comes to mind whenever I think about the topic of hope. You remember the story, I imagine. Ebenezer Scrooge, a surly old miser, is visited one Christmas Eve by three ghosts—the ghosts of Christmas Past, Present, and Future. First Scrooge goes back in time to revisit his life as a youth; some of his past Christmas Eves were quite happy and others were quite sad. Then the Ghost of Christmas Present takes him to see how the family of his employee, Bob Cratchit, is celebrating Christmas that year, and Scrooge is moved to see how the family experiences so much joy despite their challenging circumstances. Finally the Ghost of Christmas Future pulls back the curtain to show Scrooge his future, and what Scrooge sees is horribly upsetting. Not only is Scrooge dead, but the people of his community celebrate his death and mock the man he was, rather than mourn him.

The Ghost of Christmas Future doesn't speak, but Scrooge still has a question for him, a tremendously important question. Here's what he begs the ghost to tell him: "Are these visions of things that *must* be, or are they visions of things that *might* be?" That's an important question, isn't it? It's important for Scrooge, and it's important for us. But the answer Ebenezer Scrooge wants is different from the answer I want. Scrooge's hope is that these are only visions of what *might* be, because then there is still time for him to turn his life around and become a different man. But when I read what the Bible says about the future, when I read the Apostle John's vision of the heavenly kingdom in the book of Revelation, when I read about the end of my pain and the healing of my hurts, my hope is that these are visions of what *must* be.

Look at what John reveals to us about our future hope in Revelation 21: "He will wipe every tear from their eyes. There will be no more death or mourning or crying or pain, for the old order of things has passed away" (Revelation 21:4). No more death or mourning or crying or pain—that's our hope for the long haul. There is coming a day, the Bible promises us, when pain will meet its match. And the Bible gives us this assurance; these visions of the future are not visions of what *might* be; they are visions of what *will* be. John's vision of our forever future is something we can count on. It's not simply wishful thinking. It's not something we tell ourselves or others to make ourselves feel better. It's a future we can bank on.

And having that hope makes all the difference when pain has the upper hand in your life. Think about the last time you had a bad cold or a case of the flu. It was miserable, wasn't it? The coughing, the nose that won't stop running, the itchy eyes, the nausea, the achiness, and everything else that comes with it. But here's the thing—you've had colds before; you've had the flu before. And even though you were miserable, you had a very strong hope that eventually, in the not-too-distant future, you were going to get better. While you might have been discouraged by your sickness, you never felt a sense of despair.

But let's imagine you have some new pain in your life, a pain that grabs your attention and won't let go. You try taking pain-killers. You try ice and heat. You get X-rays; you have blood tests done. And while no one denies that you're in pain, no one can really explain what's causing it, much less what can be done to make it go away. Weeks go by, then months, and you're still in pain. And now you feel something else, something on top of the pain—*despair.* You knew you'd get over your cold, but this, well, you have no idea if you'll ever get over this. Or maybe it's not a physical pain that's the source of your despair; it's a broken heart, a tortured memory, a shattered relationship. But whatever your pain, your fear is this: that this might be—in the words of that old movie—"as good as it gets." And if this is really as good as it gets, then you're not sure you're going to make it.

But the Bible is very clear about this. No matter how hopeless things might seem, this is *not* as good as it gets. Someday, you will be better. And not just better than you are now—better than you've ever been, better than you could ever dream of being.

When I was in elementary school, I remember dreaming of the day when I would grow up to be big and strong and fast. I was a pretty good athlete as a little kid, but I was quite scrawny. So at night I would sometimes lie back and imagine what it might be like in ten years or so when I was 6'3", could jump over a horse, and was as fast as an NFL wide receiver. Of course, that day never came. My hopes were only hopes of what might be, not of what must be.

Now, I did get bigger and stronger and faster as time went along. But only to a point. And then one day it hit me. I didn't want to admit it, but the evidence was undeniable—not only was I not getting faster, I was getting slower. I was still in my twenties and I was already past my prime physically. As far as quickness and endurance and jumping ability, it turned out that high school was as good as it got.

But no matter how healthy you are or how much pain you may be in, the Bible wants us to understand something: *this is not as good as it gets*. The Bible has a wonderful word to describe what is ahead for all of us who follow Jesus, and that word is this— *glory*. As we come to the end of this journey on how to live with pain without becoming one, I want to look briefly at four New Testament passages which assure us that no matter how hard our present circumstances might be, we can know beyond all doubt that our future will be glorious. Knowing that and having that hope can give all who hurt the strength not just to endure but to live well no matter how dark the night might be.

Anyone who wrestles with the Christian view of pain and suffering has heard of or seen quotes from C. S. Lewis's book *The Problem of Pain*. Significantly, the last chapter of *The Problem of Pain* is simply entitled "Heaven." Lewis explains why such a chapter is necessary to make sense out of suffering when he says this: "[A] book on suffering which says nothing of heaven is leaving out almost the whole of one side of the account. Scripture and tradition habitually put the joys of heaven into the scale against the sufferings of earth, and no solution of the problem of pain which does not do so can be called a Christian one."[1]

Raised in Glory

Since we've been talking in large part about our bodies, let's start with what Bible students call the "resurrection" chapter— 1 Corinthians 15. In this chapter, the Apostle Paul addresses those who argue that there is no such thing as life after death. You may have had conversations with people who come from that point of view, people who believe that this life is all there is. But Paul says to look at the evidence. And the evidence is this—Jesus Christ not only was crucified and buried, but three days after His crucifixion, He was physically and quite literally raised back to life. In other words, says Paul, how can you say there's no life after death when so many people of that day and time saw Jesus both die and come back to life?

Then we come to verse 35, where Paul entertains another argument: "But someone will ask, 'How are the dead raised? With what kind of body will they come?'" It's a good question. It's a question a lot of us have. And here, in brief, is Paul's answer: "So it will be with the resurrection of the dead. The body that is sown is perishable, it is raised imperishable; it is sown in dishonor, it is raised in glory; it is sown in weakness, it is raised in power; it is sown a natural body, it is raised a spiritual body" (1 Corinthians 15:42–44).

A number of years ago we celebrated my mom's ninetieth birthday, and for her birthday I put together a book of pictures of her life. There were pictures of my mom as an infant and as a high schooler; pictures of her wedding day when she married my dad; pictures of her with me and my two older brothers. For some reason it's hard for a son to think this about his mother, but I have to admit that when my mom was young, she was awfully good looking. But by the time she was 95, life was very hard for Mom. She needed a walker to get around; then only a wheelchair would do. Her legs were swollen and the veins made her legs look black and blue. Just a few years ago I could still give my mom a big, strong hug and she would give me one back. At 95, she was so frail I was afraid to hug her very tightly. There were spots all over her hands and arms. She became more and more forgetful and more and more confused. And while she never liked to complain, she was quite honest when I asked her how she was doing—she hurt all the time, she said.

But my mom had a hope, a hope not merely of what might be but of what will be. Listen to how her hope is described in the book of Philippians: "But our citizenship is in heaven. And we eagerly await a Savior from there, the Lord Jesus Christ, who, by the power that enables him to bring everything under his control, will transform our lowly bodies so that they will be like his glorious body" (Philippians 3:20–21). My mom died just a handful of days after she turned 96, and the hope that sustained her for so many years is now my hope for her, that one day my mom's lowly body will be transformed so that her aged, bruised, tired body will be like Jesus's glorious body. Her body, sown in dishonor, will one day be raised in glory.

I have two brothers. Jim is in his seventies now and Dave his sixties. Once upon a time, Jim was in good shape. He was in the army and served a stint in Vietnam. But Jim has had six heart attacks in the last fifteen years. When he was in his twenties, Jim got hit by a truck while he was riding his motorcycle, and he lost part of his left leg. I will never forget sitting in the hospital with him after his leg had been amputated and watching him writhe in pain—pain he's had to manage for the rest of his life. And once upon a time, my brother Dave was an outstanding athlete, co-captain of a state championship football team and cocaptain of the wrestling team. But Dave's thyroid became so diseased a number of years ago that his thyroid crushed his trachea; he almost died from the resulting surgeries. His heart is good, but his back is his weak spot—he's had five back surgeries, with more to come. Compared to my brothers, I am—and I find this somewhat ironic—the picture of health.

But here's my hope—that what is sown in weakness will be raised in power, and what was in sown in dishonor will be raised in glory. Someday, for those who follow Jesus, our lowly bodies will be transformed so that they will be like the glorious body of our Lord. Today there may be pain and heartache and confusion and frustration. But someday pain will meet its match. Someday pain will be no more, and we will be made well in every sense of the word. Someday we will be raised in glory.

INCOMPARABLE GLORY

The Bible has a lot to say about pain. But here's what surprises me when I review many of the places where the Bible addresses pain. When I went back and looked at the main passages addressing suffering and pain, there was almost always one other word the writers used: *glory.* Let me show you what I mean.

I've quoted Romans 8 several times in this book, where Paul tells us that all of creation is in decay and subject to frustration because of the sin of mankind. He explains to us that one of the reasons for our suffering is that we live in a fallen world, that creation is broken. But notice what Paul says just before he launches into that explanation; notice the perspective he offers all of us who suffer: "Now if we are children, then we are heirs—heirs of God and co-heirs with Christ, if indeed we share in his sufferings in order that we may also share in his glory. I consider that our present sufferings are not worth comparing with the glory that will be revealed in us" (Romans 8:17–18).

Paul wants us to understand that the suffering we experience here and now is going to make our experience of glory all the sweeter. The first twenty-three winters of my life, I spent in Minnesota. One night during my last winter there, I went out to my car to drive home; it was about midnight. I got partway down the alley when I noticed I had a flat tire. In addition to the flat tire, I was stuck in an icy rut. I won't bore you with the whole story, but when I finally got the tire changed and got out of the rut over three hours later, I had three mildly frostbitten fingers. Even today when it gets cold outside, those three fingers turn white and as hard as rocks. It was a miserable night.

Two months after that I moved to California to finish up seminary in San Diego. I immediately drove to the beach. I sat there in my Plymouth Volare station wagon with its wood paneling on the side (a truly ugly car) for the better part of two hours just staring at the setting sun, listening to the waves, and soaking up the warmth. It was glorious! And what made that moment all the more glorious for me was the fact that just a week earlier I was still shoveling snow back in Minnesota. The "suffering" I went through back there made the glory of a San Diego sunset on the beach all the better.

My stepfather, Kenny, was the gentlest and most content man

I've ever known. In the twenty-five years he was married to my mom before he passed away at the age of 88, I never once heard him complain. When I asked him about it, he explained that it went back to when he was in Italy during World War II, serving in the army. His platoon spent some frigid winter nights holed up in the ice and snow, taking enemy fire throughout. It was miserable and it was terrifying. Kenny had many hours to talk to God about his situation, and during that time he made God a promise—if he got out of the cold and the shelling alive, he would never complain again.

Kenny survived, with all his body parts functioning. And the suffering he went through during World War II made any inconvenience he experienced thereafter so inconsequential that he never had reason to complain again.

Paul wants us to understand that our present sufferings will only make our future glory all the sweeter. And he wants us to focus on something else: there's no comparison between the two. Let me see if I can illustrate what "no comparison" means. My wife's car is a 2007 black Honda Civic. You've probably noticed that there are a lot of black cars on the road; my Hyundai Sonata is also black. A number of times over the years we've entered the Safeway parking lot to get into Brenda's car and she's walked up to a black BMW or a black Mercedes and tried to open the door, thinking it was her Honda Civic. Our thoroughly embarrassed son would say, "Mom, that's not your car!" And Brenda would reply, "How can you tell? They're both black." Ryan and I are thinking, "There's no comparison between your Civic and this BMW." But Brenda is thinking, "They're both black, they both have four doors, and they pretty much have the same shape." And do you know what? To a degree, she's right. One is much nicer and much more expensive than the other, but there's still a comparison to be made.

But let me ask you this—would you ever compare a Honda Civic, with 140 hp, to a solid rocket booster, the kind used for years to launch the shuttle into space? To launch a space shuttle requires, I am told, 81 million hp. Even if they painted it black and put four doors on it, you'd never confuse a Civic for a rocket. There's no comparison. And that, Paul tells us, is the difference between our present sufferings and our future glory. Here is our hope for the long haul, and it is very sure: the glory waiting for us will leave our pain and suffering in the dust.

ETERNAL GLORY

Not only is this glory we are promised an incomparable glory, but it will also be an *eternal glory*. Let's go back to another key New Testament passage on pain and suffering—2 Corinthians 4. Here's what Paul writes:

> Therefore, we do not lose heart. Though outwardly we are wasting away, yet inwardly we are being renewed day by day. For our light and momentary troubles are achieving for us an eternal glory that far outweighs them all. So we fix our eyes not on what is seen, but on what is unseen, since what is seen is temporary, but what is unseen is eternal (2 Corinthians 4:16–18).

I imagine there are quite a lot of folk around the globe who might want to take issue with Paul's assessment of our troubles as "light and momentary." In the book *The Insanity of God,* Nik

Ripken—who left Kentucky with his young wife to spend six years as missionaries and aid workers in Somalia—describes the horrific suffering he saw in that part of the world, suffering fairly labeled "insane."[2] And I imagine every one of us could tell a tale of suffering we've seen ourselves, if not experienced ourselves, that we would argue was anything but light and momentary. Nick Vujicic was born without any arms or legs—he's an incredibly positive person who has accomplished exceptional things, but that kind of disability strikes me as something more than light and momentary.[3] A teenage girl we knew years ago woke up from a fairly routine surgery to discover she couldn't swallow . . . ever again. How's that momentary?

But Paul, no stranger to suffering himself, encourages us to focus on the truly long haul, on eternity. Compared to eternity, Paul reminds us, anything we suffer here on this earth is merely momentary. Think of it like this. Have you noticed that infants aren't very patient? When an infant is hungry, she needs to be fed and she needs to be fed *now* or she's going to make your life miserable. But you don't act that way, do you? At least I hope you don't. At about ten in the morning you might think, "I'm getting a little hungry." But you don't fall to the ground in a puddle of tears and demand that your boss bring you food. You think, "Two more hours, and then I can have some lunch." To the infant, a minute is too long; to you, a minute is a mere moment.

One day, the Bible tells us, we will look back on our suffering—no matter how truly miserable it may well have been—and it will seem to us to have lasted a mere moment, a blink of the eye. And Paul challenges us to handle our pain here and now by fixing our eyes not on the here and now but on the then and there, on our forever future, when pain and suffering are swallowed up by eternal glory.

When I was learning to drive, my father taught me an important principle: two bodies cannot occupy the same space at the same time. If two vehicles were to collide, the heavier one would displace the lighter one. Since I was driving a Ford Pinto at the time, I had no trouble getting his point.

In the Bible, the Hebrew word for *glory* originally meant "weight" or "heaviness."[4] That same idea comes through in the New Testament as well, as we've already seen. As Paul says it, "For our light and momentary troubles are achieving for us an eternal glory that far outweighs them all" (2 Corinthians 4:17). In other words, someday glory is going to displace pain; glory is going to inhabit the space that pain occupied in our lives. And the better news? The glory will never end.

JOYFUL GLORY

Finally, the Bible describes the glory waiting for us at the proverbial end of the rainbow as a *joyful glory*. Look at what the Apostle Peter tells us: "Dear friends, do not be surprised at the fiery ordeal that has come on you to test you, as though something strange were happening to you. But rejoice inasmuch as you participate in the sufferings of Christ, so that you may be overjoyed when his glory is revealed" (1 Peter 4:12–13). In one of the opening sentences of that same letter, Peter writes that even though we now "suffer grief in all kinds of trials," the day is coming when we will be filled with an "inexpressible and glorious joy" (1 Peter 1:6, 8).

When our three kids were fairly young, our family took a trip to Yosemite, truly one of the most beautiful places on earth. We were all together near the campground store. Brenda decided to go into the store to get some supplies for the short hike we planned, and I went on ahead to get the lay of the land. I was quite sure that all three kids—Stephanie, age 7; Ryan, age 4; and Kelsey, age 2—went with their mom, while Brenda was quite sure that Ryan was with me. Long story short, Ryan got separated from us (actually, from me, as it turned out). And you can imagine the panic and dread that washed over us when we realized that our young son was lost in this sea of people. We ran from place to place, person to person, calling out Ryan's name, doing our best—frankly—to keep from throwing up.

I finally calmed down enough to think, "Okay, if I were in Ryan's shoes, where would I have gone?" I realize that doesn't always work, but on this occasion it did. About a football field away I saw our little boy, sitting by a tree, feeling very lost and hoping to be found. And do you want to guess what I felt when I saw him? "Inexpressible and glorious joy"!

Now imagine your first glimpse of "glory." Imagine how you will feel when you see the face of Jesus as He welcomes you to your eternal home. Imagine how you will feel as you look around and see those loved ones who preceded you to glory and it dawns on you that you will never be separated again. Imagine how you will feel when it occurs to you that your pain is gone, that you are stronger and better than you ever dreamed possible, and that you know you will never suffer for even a second for the rest of eternity. Never again will you be sad or disappointed or ashamed. No more headaches, no more backaches, no more bruises, no more disease . . . no more pain. You can guess what you will feel—inexpressible and glorious joy!

The Bible tells us this: "Since, then, you have been raised with Christ, set your hearts on things above, where Christ is, seated at the right hand of God" (Colossians 3:1). If we want to live with our pain without becoming one, that's exactly what we need to do, to set our hearts on the glory that will be ours for eternity. Now maybe that sounds a bit naive, a bit simplistic. Does dreaming about the by and by really help us handle the here and now? Joni Eareckson Tada thinks so. Joni, you'll recall, has been a quadriplegic since 1967. Yet in her books, Joni often writes that she thinks about heaven every day . . . and that it is the hope of heaven that gives her the courage she needs to get through another day of frustration, limitation, and pain. Perhaps that sentiment is best expressed in a song written for her by Nancy Honeytree called "Joni's Waltz."[5] In the song, Joni explains that while she is destined to spend her earthly lifetime in a wheelchair, she can live without despair because her suffering makes heaven nearer to her. Looking past her pain, she looks forward with great joy to the day when she stands by Jesus's side and he invites her to dance. And, she concludes, their endless romance will be worth all the tears she's cried.

Pain is a drain—emotionally, physically, and spiritually. Living with pain can sometimes feel like a hard workout at the gym or a long day at work; it leaves you exhausted and spent. Shedding tears—which can at times be particularly therapeutic—can also be tremendously draining. When you're physically drained, you know you need to rehydrate. You give your body the water, sodium, sugar, and potassium it needs to recuperate and function well (I drink a sports drink because it gives me the illusion that I'm still an athlete). And when you're drained by pain, you similarly need something to fill you up and refresh you.

Of course, there's no sports drink on the market that restores us when our souls are drained by pain. But hope can . . . hope in the God who has promised that after we suffer for a little while, He will restore us and make us strong. Hope that God will do for us what He has said He will do—put an end to our pain, heal our hurts, redeem our suffering, and replace our grief with glory. One day our pain will meet its match, and our tears will be swallowed up by inexpressible and glorious joy. There's hope for the long haul, and His name is Jesus.

CHAPTER ONE

1. Salynn Boyles, "100 Million Americans Have Chronic Pain," *WebMD Health News* (June 29, 2011): http://www.webmd.com/pain-management/news/20110629/100-million-americans-have-chronic-pain#1; also American Academy of Pain Medicine, "AAPM Facts and Figures on Pain" (April 24, 2017): http://www.painmed.org/patientcenter/facts-on-pain/; Institute of Medicine (US) Committee on Advancing Pain Research, Care, and Education, *Relieving Pain in America: A Blueprint for Transforming Prevention, Care, Education and Research* (Washington, DC: National Academies Press, 2011), 5; The U.S. Pain Foundation at http://learnaboutyourpain.com/.

2. Holly Fletcher, "There Are More Opioid Prescriptions than There Are People in Tennessee," *The Tennessean* (September 19, 2016): http://www.tennessean.com/story/news/health/2016/09/19/there-more-opioid-prescriptions-than-people-tennessee/90358404/.

3. Northwestern University, "Chronic Back Pain Shrinks 'Thinking Parts' of Brain" research study (November 23, 2004): www.northwestern.edu/newscenter/stories/2004/11/chronic.html.

4. Mandy Oaklander, "The Science of Crying," *Time Magazine* (March 16, 2016).

5. Jacob Rascon, "Making a Difference," *NBC Nightly News* (July 23, 2014): https://archive.org/details/KNTV_20140724_003000_NBC_Nightly_News/start/1620/end/1680.

6. Timothy Keller, *Walking with God through Pain and Suffering* (New York: Dutton, 2013), 203.

CHAPTER TWO

1. Cindy Wooden, "Pope, with Fellow Jesuits, Prays for 'Grace of Shame,' Humility," *Catholic News Service* (July 31, 2013): http://www.catholicnews.com/services/englishnews/2013/pope-with-fellow-jesuits-prays-for-grace-of-shame-humility-cns-1303309.cfm.

2. Guy Winch, "The Surprising Upside of Guilt and Shame," *The Squeaky Wheel* blog, *Psychology Today* (March 7, 2015): https://www.psychologytoday.com/blog/the-squeaky-wheel/201503/the-surprising-upside-guilt-and-shame.

3. The Free Dictionary, "Pain Management" (April 24, 2017): http://medical-dictionary.thefreedictionary.com/pain+management.

4. BoneSmart, "How Successful Is Hip Replacement Surgery?" *BoneSmart.org* (April 24, 2017): http://bonesmart.org/hip/how-successful-is-hip-replacement-surgery/.

5. Bible Hub, "Katartizó," *BibleHub.org* (April 24, 2017): http://biblehub.com/greek/2675.htm.

CHAPTER FOUR

1. Bob Costas, Interview of Mickey Mantle (March 1994): https://www.youtube.com/watch?v=Hm_Ybn4JMxM.

2. Derek Terry, "After Years of Addiction and Tragedy, Former Star Recruit Zeke Pike Is Finding His Way Back," *Sports Illustrated* (December 26, 2016): http://www.si.com /college-football/2016/12/26/zeke-pike-auburn-tigers-louisville-cardinals.

3. A. J. Perez, "The Chicago Cubs' Billy Goat Curse, Explained," *USA Today* (October 25, 2016): http://www.usatoday.com/story/sports/mlb/2016/10/25/chicago-cubs-billy -goat-curse-explained/92715898/.

4. DominoDomain, "World Record History," *DominoDomain.org* (April 24, 2017): http:// www.dominodomain.com/fan-area/domino-day/world-record-history/.

CHAPTER FIVE

1. Lewis B. Smedes, *The Art of Forgiving* (Nashville, TN: Moorings, 1996), 57.

2. Timothy Keller, *Walking with God through Pain and Suffering* (New York: Dutton, 2013), 260.

3. Ibid., 140–141. Timothy Keller explains it like this, noting that the biblical doctrine of God's sovereignty is sometimes labeled "compatibilism." "The Bible teaches that God is completely in control of what happens in history and yet He exercises that control in such a way that human beings are responsible for their freely chosen actions and the results of those actions . . . . To put it most practically and vividly—if a man robs a bank, that moral evil is fully his responsibility, though it is also part of God's plan. . . . Ultimately, there are no accidents. His plan also includes bad things."

4. Leonard Sweet, *Soul Salsa,* (Grand Rapids, MI: Zondervan, 2000).

5. Douglas Groothius, "Bedeviled by My Wife's Dementia," *Christianity Today* (October 2015): http://www.christianitytoday.com/ct/2015/november/bedeviled-by-my-wifes -dementia.html.

6. Steve Hartman, "Innocent Man Ends Up Pals with Crooked Cop That Framed Him," *CBS News* (April 15, 2016): http://www.cbsnews.com/news/on-the-road-innocent -michigan-man-ends-up-working-alongside-crooked-cop-that-locked-him/.

7. Robert Hull, producer, "Kelly Putty: Rape Victim Forgives Attackers," *The 700 Club* (April 24, 2017): http://www1.cbn.com/700club/ kelly-putty-rape-victim-forgives-attackers.

8. Allyson R. Quinn, "The Fruit of Forgiveness," *Prison Fellowship* (April 9, 2011): https://www.prisonfellowship.org/2011/04/the-fruit-of-forgiveness/.

9. Kelly and Shane Putty's child-advocacy organization: http://ordinaryhero.org/.

10. Quinn, "The Fruit of Forgiveness."

11. Kathryn Watterson, *Not by the Sword: How a Cantor and His Family Transformed a Klansman* (Boston: Northeastern University Press, 2001).

CHAPTER SIX

1. Timothy Keller, *Walking with God through Pain and Suffering* (New York: Dutton, 2013), 17.

2. Ibid., 18–20.

3. Jesus also makes the point in Luke 13:1–5 that there are times when bad things happen to people for reasons that defy an easy explanation and that it's often inappropriate to suggest that a person's suffering is caused by their sin: "Or those eighteen who died when the tower in Siloam fell on them—do you think they were more guilty than all the others living in Jerusalem? I tell you, no!" (Luke 13:4–5 NIV).
4. Philip Yancey, *The Question That Never Goes Away: Why?* (Grand Rapids, MI: Zondervan, 2013).
5. Keller, *Walking with God*, 281.
6. Douglas Groothius, "Bedeviled by My Wife's Dementia," *Christianity Today* (October 2015): http://www.christianitytoday.com/ct/2015/november/bedeviled-by-my-wifes-dementia.html.
7. Yancey, *The Question.*.
8. Katie Jo Ramsey, "The Truth About Living with an Invisible Illness," *Christianity Today* (July 2016): http://www.christianitytoday.com/women/2016/july/truth-about-living-with-invisible-illness.html.
9. Raymond F. Collins, *1 and 2 Timothy and Titus: A Commentary* (Louisville, KY: Westminster John Knox Press, 2002), 201.
10. Joni Eareckson Tada and Steven Estes, *A Step Further* (Grand Rapids, MI: Zondervan, 1978), 97.

CHAPTER SEVEN
1. The Free Dictionary, "Patient" (April 24, 2017): http://www.thefreedictionary.com/patient.
2. C. S. Lewis, *The Problem of Pain,* (New York: McMillan, 1962), 102.
3. BibleHub, "Koinónia," *BibleHub.org* (April 24, 2017): http://biblehub.com/greek/2842.htm.
4. Laura Thomas, "A Stroke Freed Me from Fleeting Beauty," *Christianity Today* (February 19, 2017): http://www.christianitytoday.com/women/2017/february/stroke-freed-me-from-fleeting-beauty.html.
5. Katherine and Jay Wolf's disability ministry, Hope Heals:www.hopeheals.com.

CHAPTER EIGHT
1. Randy Alcorn, *If God Is Good,*(Colorado Springs: Multnomah, 2009), 136.
2. Joni Eareckson Tada and Steven Estes, *When God Weeps: Why Our Sufferings Matter to the Almighty* (Grand Rapids, MI: Zondervan, 1997), 84.
3. James Dobson, *When God Doesn't Make Sense* (Wheaton, IL: Tyndale, 1993), 60–62.
4. Edith Schaeffer, *Affliction* (Old Tappan, NJ: Revell, 1978), 78–81.
5. Tada and Estes echo this point in *When God Weeps,* 106–108.
6. God has not clearly revealed to me that this pain is "just plain evil," and I can't say with complete certainty that it is. But I certainly have my suspicions.
7. Lady Gaga, "Applause" (April 24, 2017): http://www.azlyrics.com/lyrics/ladygaga/applause.html.

ENDNOTES

8. Bible Hub, "Sunagónizomai," *BibleHub.org* (April 24, 2017): http://biblehub.com /greek/4865.htm.
9. The Famous People, "Pope John Paul II," *Thefamouspeople.com* (April 24, 2017): http:// www.thefamouspeople.com/profiles/pope-john-paul-ii-81.php.
10. Christopher Kaczor, "A Pope's Answer to the Problem of Pain," *Catholic Answers Magazine* (November 21, 2011): https://www.catholic.com/magazine/ print-edition/a-popes-answer-to-the-problem-of-pain.
11. Kaczor, "A Pope's Answer to the Problem of Pain."
12. Earnest Ogbozor, "Love and Forgiveness in Governance,"*BeyondIntractability.org* (April 25, 2017): http://www.beyondintractability.org/lfg/exemplars/jpaul.
13. Pope John Paul II, *"Salvifici Doloris"* (February 11, 1984): http://w2.vatican.va/content /john-paul-ii/en/apost_letters/1984/documents/hf_jp-ii_apl_11021984_salvifici -doloris.html.

CHAPTER NINE

1. Tenth Avenue North (Jason Ingram, Jeff Owen, and Mike Donehey), "Worn," *"The Struggle,"* copyright song/ATV Music Publishing LLC (2012).
2. Ashley Hayes, "Loneliness: Five Things You May Not Know," *CNN.com* (November 26, 2014): http://www.cnn.com/2014/02/19/health/lonely-research/.
3. Tenth Avenue North, "Worn."

CHAPTER TEN

1. Rick Warren, "The Most Important Interview I've Ever Done" (September 13, 2013): http://pastors.com/piers/#; "CNN Transcripts," *Piers Morgan Live, CNN.com* (April 25, 2017): http://transcripts.cnn.com/TRANSCRIPTS/1309/17/pmt.01.html.
2. Max Lucado, *Just Like Jesus* (Nashville, TN: Thomas Nelson, 1998).
3. U.S. Pain Foundation: https://www.uspainfoundation.org/.
4. Ibid, https://www.uspainfoundation.org/programs/.
5. Catherine Woodiwiss,"A New Normal: Ten Things I've Learned About Trauma," *Sojourners Magazine* (January 13, 2014): https://sojo.net/articles/new-normal-ten -things-ive-learned-about-trauma.

CHAPTER ELEVEN

1. U.S. Pain Foundation, "Complementary Therapies" *U.S. Pain Foundation* (April 25, 2017): https://www.uspainfoundation.org/resources-2/complementary-therapies/.
2. Ibid, "Crystal Therapy."
3. Kent M. Keith, "The Paradoxical Commandments" (1968): http://www. paradoxicalcommandments.com/.
4. John Ortberg, *Soul Keeping: Caring for the Most Important Part of You* (Grand Rapids, MI: Zondervan, 2014), 40.

CHAPTER TWELVE

1. C. S. Lewis, *The Problem of Pain* (New York: McMillan, 1962), 144.
2. Nik Ripken and Gregg Lewis, *The Insanity of God: A True Story of Faith Resurrected* (Nashville, TN: B&H, 2013).
3. Nick Vujicic, *Life without Limits: Inspiration for a Ridiculously Good Life* (Colorado Springs: WaterBrook, 2010).
4. Christian Apologetics and Research Ministry, Dictionary of Theology, "Glory," *CARM* (April 27, 2017): https://carm.org/dictionary-glory.
5. Nancy Honeytree, "Joni's Waltz," *Heaven: Your Real Home,* by Joni Eareckson Tada (Grand Rapids, MI: Zondervan, 1995), 11.

ABOUT THE AUTHOR

Craig Selness was born and raised in Minnesota before moving to California in 1979, where he has lived ever since. He received his B.A. from the University of Minnesota in 1976, his Master of Divinity degree from Bethel Seminary in St. Paul, Minnesota in 1979, his M.A. in Pastoral Counseling from Santa Clara University in 1982, and his J.D. from the University of California, Berkeley in 1985.

Craig served as the assistant pastor of Willow Glen Baptist Church in San Jose from 1979 to 1984, and during that time authored two books published by Victor Books: *There's More To Life!* and *When Your Mountain Won't Move*. Beginning in 1985 Craig worked as an employment lawyer in the Silicon Valley, full-time until 1997 and part-time from 1997 until 2001.

In 1992 Craig and his wife Brenda started Cornerstone Community Church, a church affiliated with Converge Worldwide; Craig was the senior pastor of Cornerstone for 23 years. In February of 2016 Cornerstone merged with Menlo Church San Jose, where Craig serves as the Pastor of Community Life.

Craig married Brenda in 1980; Brenda has managed a law firm in San Jose for over 32 years. Together they have three grown children—Stephanie, Ryan, and Kelsey. Stephanie and her husband, Scott, have two children.

**IF YOU ENJOYED THIS BOOK, WILL YOU CONSIDER
SHARING THE MESSAGE WITH OTHERS?**

Mention the book in a blog post or through Facebook, Twitter, Pinterest, or upload a picture through Instagram.

Recommend this book to those in your small group, book club, workplace, and classes.

Head over to facebook.com/worthypublishing, "LIKE" the page, and post a comment as to what you enjoyed the most.

Tweet "I recommend reading #LivingWithPain by @cselness // @worthypub"

Pick up a copy for someone you know who would be challenged and encouraged by this message.

Write a book review online.

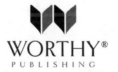

Visit us at worthypublishing.com

twitter.com/worthypub

worthypub.tumblr.com

facebook.com/worthypublishing

pinterest.com/worthypub

instagram.com/worthypub

youtube.com/worthypublishing